Clinical Cases in Dermatology

Series Editor
Robert A. Norman
Tampa, FL, USA

This series of concise practical guides is designed to facilitate the clinical decision-making process by reviewing a number of cases and defining the various diagnostic and management decisions open to clinicians.

Each title is illustrated and diverse in scope, enabling the reader to obtain relevant clinical information regarding both standard and unusual cases in a rapid, easy to digest format. Each focuses on one disease or patient group, and includes common cases to allow readers to know they are doing things right if they follow the case guidelines.

More information about this series at http://link.springer.com/series/10473

Anna Waśkiel-Burnat • Roxanna Sadoughifar
Torello M. Lotti • Lidia Rudnicka

Editors

Clinical Cases in Hair Disorders

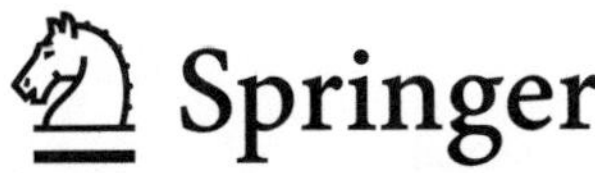

Editors
Anna Waśkiel-Burnat
Dermatology
Medical University of Warsaw
Warsaw, Poland

Roxanna Sadoughifar
Dermatology
Marconi University
Rome, Roma, Italy

Torello M. Lotti
Dermatology
University of Rome "G.Marconi"
Rome, Roma, Italy

Lidia Rudnicka
Dermatology
Medical University of Warsaw
Warsaw, Poland

ISSN 2730-6178 ISSN 2730-6186 (electronic)
Clinical Cases in Dermatology
ISBN 978-3-030-93422-4 ISBN 978-3-030-93423-1 (eBook)
https://doi.org/10.1007/978-3-030-93423-1

This Springer imprint is published by the registered company Springer Nature Switzerland AG
The registered company address is: Gewerbestrasse 11, 6330 Cham, Switzerland

Contents

Chapter 1
19-Year-Old Woman with Short, Spiky, Brittle Hair

Aleksandra Kaczyńska-Trzpil, Agnieszka Gradzińska, and Adriana Rakowska

A 19-year-old woman was admitted to the Department of Dermatology due to generalized red scaly patches on the skin and short, dry, spiky hair. The patient reported coexisted itch. The lesions persisted from the birth. Gastroesophageal reflux and blood-mixed mucoid stool at the age of three months were observed. Allergy to cow's milk, egg, peanuts and soya was diagnosed. The patient was previously treated with topical corticosteroids and pimecrolimus with no significant improvement. The parents of the patients were healthy and unrelated.

A physical examination revealed erythroderma with coexisted scaling. Moreover, sparse and short brittle hair were observed (Fig. 1.1). On trichoscopy, trichorrhexis invaginata, matchstick and golf tee hairs were detected (Fig. 1.2).

Laboratory tests revealed eosinophilia (4.24×10^3/ml with normal range 0–0.5×10^3/ml) and increased IgE level (2500 IU/ml with normal range: 0–100 IU/ml).

Based on the case description and the photographs, what is your diagnosis?

Differential Diagnoses

1. Netherton syndrome.
2. Atopic dermatitis.
3. Psoriasis.
4. Seborrheic dermatitis.

A. Kaczyńska-Trzpil (✉) · A. Gradzińska · A. Rakowska
Department of Dermatology, Medical University of Warsaw, Warsaw, Poland
e-mail: adriana.rakowska@wum.edu.pl

A. Waśkiel-Burnat et al. (eds.), *Clinical Cases in Hair Disorders*, Clinical Cases in Dermatology, https://doi.org/10.1007/978-3-030-93423-1_1

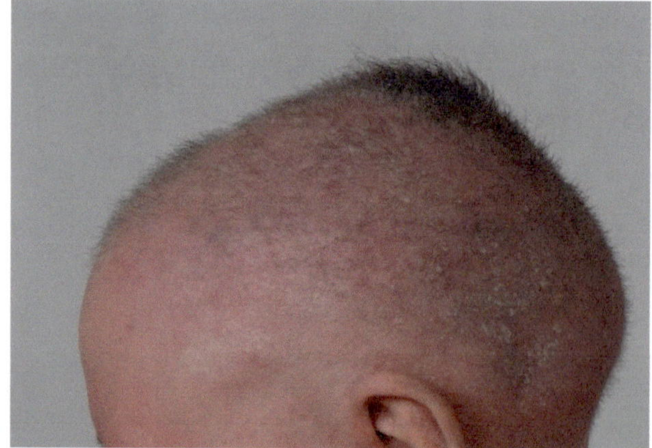

Fig. 1.1 A 19-year-old woman with red, scaly patches on the scalp and dry, spiky hair

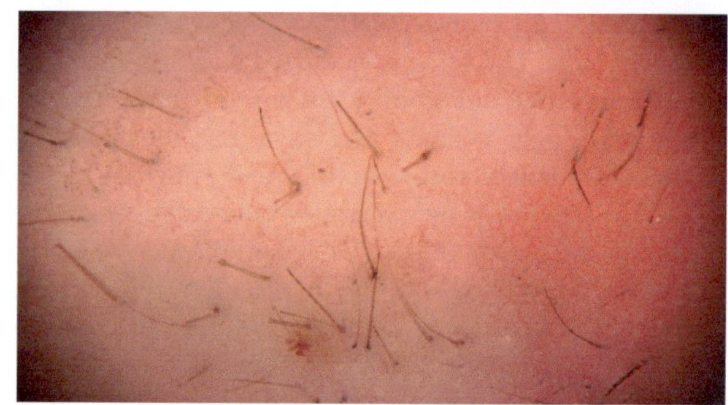

Fig. 1.2 Trichoscopy shows trichorrhexis invaginata, matchstick and golf tee hairs (×20)

Diagnosis

Netherton syndrome.

Discussion

Netherton syndrome is a rare autosomal recessive genodermatosis, characterized by a triad of congenital ichthyosiform erythroderma or ichthyosis linearis circumflexa, hair shaft abnormalities, and atopic diathesis (elevated serum IgE). The condition affects 1 per 200,000 newborns [1]. Netherton syndrome is caused by loss-of-function mutations in the serine protease inhibitor (SPINK5) on chromosome 5q32 which encodes for the serine protease inhibitor LEKTI. It results in an increased activity of epidermal proteases which cause premature desquamation of the stratum corneum and impairment of the skin barrier. Congenital ichthyosiform erythro-derma is the generalized erythroderma and desquamation present at birth. It evolves into a migratory, erythematous, serpiginous patches with double-edged scales at the periphery. This ichthyosis linearis circumflexa waxes and wanes throughout the patient's life and is associated with pruritus [1–3]. Concomitant atopic diathesis contributes to many food allergies, severe enteropathy, eosinophilic oesophagitis, eosinophilic colitis leading to diarrhea, growth retardation, failure to thrive, mental retardation, and hypoalbuminemia. Allergic rhinitis, asthma, urticaria and angioedema may occur. IgE levels are significantly elevated and hypereosinophilia is present. In severe generalized forms patients, especially young infants, are prone to systemic complications due to impairment of thermoregulation and fluid loss and may develop hypothermia, hypernatremic dehydration, seizures, and renal failure. Because of the defective skin barrier, recurrent bacterial skin infections are common [4–7]. In patients with Netherton syndrome hair shaft abnormalities are observed. The hairs are sparse, short, dry, and brittle. Trichoscopy reveals trichorrhexis invaginata ("bamboo hair"), seen as nodules along hair shaft in low-magnification and invagination of distal part into proximal part of hair shaft (resembling ball in cup) in high-magnification. As this feature is pathognomonic for Netherton syndrome, it is sufficient to confirm the diagnosis. Other trichoscopic findings of Netherton syndrome are golf tee hairs and matchstick hairs [7]. The most common histopathological finding of the condition is psoriasiform epidermal hyperplasia. Other features include compact parakeratosis with large nuclei, subcorneum or intracorneum splitting, presence of clear cells in the upper epidermis or stratum corneum, dyskeratosis, dermal infiltrate with neutrophils and/or eosinophils, and dilated blood vessels in the superficial dermis. Immunohistochemistry staining shows *LEKTI* deficiency in epidermis [4, 8]. Genetic tests may be performed to confirm the diagnosis. There is no satisfactory treatment currently available for Netherton syndrome. Topical corticosteroids, topical calcineurin inhibitors, topical retinoids, narrowband ultraviolet B phototherapy, psoralen and ultraviolet irradiation, and oral acitretin are therapeutic options. In severe cases, intravenous immunoglobulin and anti-TNF may be helpful.

Netherton syndrome needs to be distinguished from atopic dermatitis, psoriasis and seborrheic dermatitis.

Atopic dermatitis is one of the most prevalent skin disorders. It usually occurs during the first year of life. The lesions presents three months after the birth. Acute lesions are characterized by intensely pruritic erythematous papules and vesicles with exudation and crusting, whereas subacute or chronic lesions present as dry, scaly, or excoriated erythematous papules. Skin thickening from chronic scratching (lichenification) and fissuring may develop over time. In infants, the skin lesions localized on the extensor surfaces, cheeks and scalp. There is usually sparing of the diaper area. In older children and adults, the flexor surfaces are mainly involved. No hair shaft abnormalities are present [1, 4].

Psoriasis is an uncommon condition in young infants. It is characterized by the presence of red, thickened plaques with silver-white scale. The condition affects mainly the extensor surface of elbows and knees, the scalp, and lower back. Erythroderma may occur. No hair shaft abnormalities are presented and joint involvement may occur [4].

Seborrheic dermatitis is a chronic inflammatory dermatologic condition that commonly occurs in infants (usually within the first three months of life). It presents as well-delimited erythematous plaques with greasy-looking, yellowish scales. The scalp is most commonly affected, however the disease can appear also on the other body areas such as the face, chest, back, axilla, and groin [5, 6]. Erythroderma may occur. No hair shaft abnormalities are presented. Seborrheic dermatitis is characterized by a seasonal pattern, presenting more frequently during winter, and usually improving during summer [2, 8].

Based on the clinical presentation and trichoscopic findings, the patient was diagnosed with Netherton syndrome. Psoralen and ultraviolet A therapy was recommended.

Key Points
- Netherton syndrome is a rare genetic disease characterized by a triad of congenital ichthyosiform erythroderma or ichthyosis linearis circumflexa, hair shaft abnormalities, and atopic diathesis (elevated serum IgE)
- In patients with Netherton syndome sparse, short, dry, and brittle hair are observed
- Trichorrhexis invaginata is pathognomonic feature of Netherton syndrome

References

1. Zhang Z, Pan C, Wei R, Li H, Yang Y, Chen J, Li M, Yao Z. Netherton syndrome caused by compound heterozygous mutation, c.80A>G mutation in SPINK5 and large-sized genomic deletion mutation, and successful treatment of intravenous immunoglobulin. Mol Genet Genomic Med. 2021 Jan 16;9(3):e1600.
2. Chiticariu E, Hohl D. Netherton syndrome: insights into pathogenesis and clinical implications. J Invest Dermatol. 2020;140(6):1129–30.
3. Gouin O, Barbieux C, Leturcq F, Bonnet des Claustres M, Petrova E, Hovnanian A. Transgenic Kallikrein 14 mice display major hair shaft defects associated with Desmoglein 3 and 4 degradation, abnormal epidermal differentiation, and IL-36 signature. J Invest Dermatol. 2020;140(6):1184–94.
4. Raghunath M, Tontsidou L, Oji V, Aufenvenne K, Schürmeyer-Horst F, Jayakumar A, Ständer H, Smolle J, Clayman GL, Traupe H. SPINK5 and Netherton syndrome: novel mutations, demonstration of missing LEKTI, and differential expression of transglutaminases. J Invest Dermatol. 2004;123(3):474–83.
5. Kilic G, Guler N, Ones U, Tamay Z, Guzel P. Netherton syndrome: report of identical twins presenting with severe atopic dermatitis. Eur J Pediatr. 2006;165(9):594–7.
6. Hannula-Jouppi K, Laasanen SL, Ilander M, Furio L, Tuomiranta M, Marttila R, Jeskanen L, Häyry V, Kanerva M, Kivirikko S, Tuomi ML, Heikkilä H, Mustjoki S, Hovnanian A, Ranki A. Intrafamily and interfamilial phenotype variation and immature immunity in patients with Netherton syndrome and Finnish SPINK5 founder mutation. JAMA Dermatol. 2016;152(4):435–42.
7. Rudnicka L, Olszewska M, Waśkiel A, Rakowska A. Trichoscopy in hair shaft disorders. Dermatol Clin. 2018;36(4):421–30.
8. Leclerc-Mercier S, Bodemer C, Furio L, Hadj-Rabia S, de Peufeilhoux L, Weibel L, Bursztejn AC, Bourrat E, Ortonne N, Molina TJ, Hovnanian A, Fraitag S. Skin biopsy in Netherton syndrome: a histological review of a large series and new findings. Am J Dermatopathol. 2016;38(2):83–91.

Chapter 2
A 14-Year-Old Boy with Hair Loss and Scaling on the Scalp

Nkechi Anne Enechukwu, Esther Ngozi Umeadi, Ogochukwu Ifeanyi Ezejiofor, and Adebola Olufunmilayo Ogunbiyi

A 14-year-old boy presented with an eight-year history of recurrent, focal scaling on the scalp associated with hair loss. He also complained of itching. The patient denied having domestic animals. No family history of similar lesions was reported.

A physical examination revealed multiple areas of scaly patches with hair loss (Fig. 2.1). On dry trichoscopy diffuse perifollicular and interfollicular yellowish-white scaling with hair casts, broken hairs and corkscrew hairs were observed (Fig. 2.2). Trichoscopy with immersion fluid showed multiple black dots, broken hairs, comma, corkscrew, i- and z-hairs (Fig. 2.3).

Based on the case description and the photographs, what is your diagnosis?

Differential Diagnoses

1. Tinea capitis.
2. Seborrheic dermatitis.
3. Alopecia areata.
4. Psoriasis.

N. A. Enechukwu (✉) · O. I. Ezejiofor
Dermatology and Venereology Unit, Department of Internal Medicine, Faculty of Medicine, Nnamdi Azikiwe University, Nnewi Campus, Anambra, Nigeria
e-mail: na.enechukwu@unizik.edu.ng

E. N. Umeadi
Department of Pediatrics, Nnamdi Azikiwe University, Nnewi, Anambra, Nigeria
e-mail: en.umeadi@unizik.edu.ng

A. O. Ogunbiyi
Department of Medicine, College of Medicine, University of Ibadan, Ibadan, Oyo, Nigeria

A. Waśkiel-Burnat et al. (eds.), *Clinical Cases in Hair Disorders*, Clinical Cases in Dermatology, https://doi.org/10.1007/978-3-030-93423-1_2

Fig. 2.1 A 14-year-old boy with multiple areas of scaly patches and hair loss

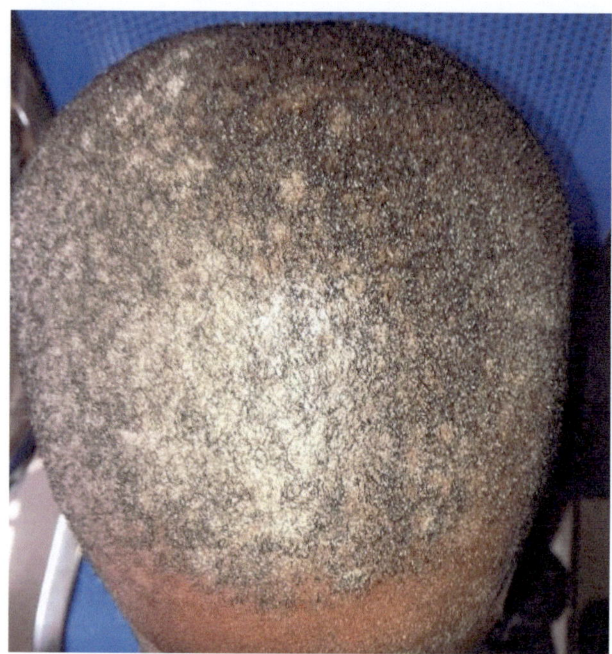

Fig. 2.2 Dry trichoscopy shows diffuse perifollicular and interfollicular yellowish-white scaling with hair casts (×40)

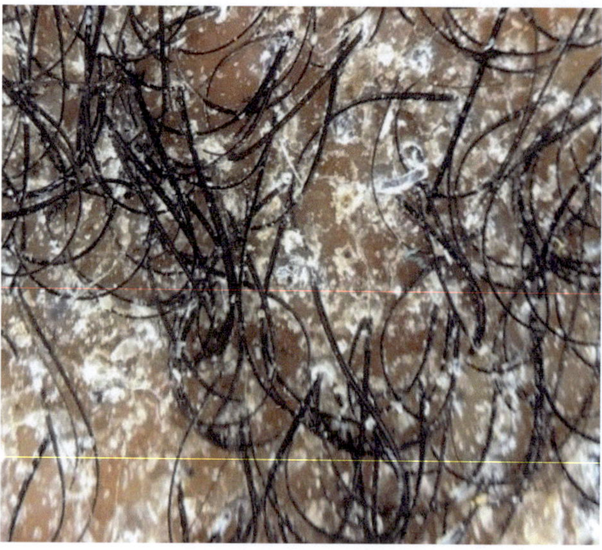

Fig. 2.3 Trichoscopy with immersion fluid black dots, broken hairs and comma hairs (×40)

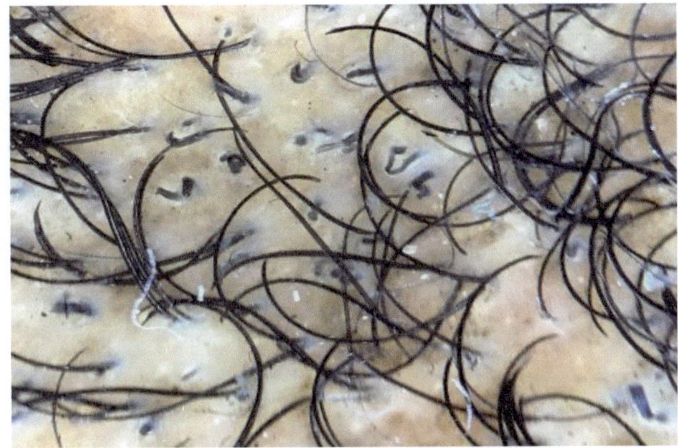

Diagnosis

Tinea capitis.

Discussion

Tinea capitis is a dermatophytosis of the scalp. It is caused by *Microsporum* and *Trichophyton* species. Human, animal or soil contact may be the source of all types of tinea capitis. The disease is most commonly observed in children between three and seven years of age. Adults (especially elderly individuals) may be occasionally affected [1]. Based on the pattern of invasion of the hair shaft, tinea capitis is classified as follow: endothrix, with the presence of multiple arthroconidia within the hair shaft; favus, with the presence of hyphae within the hair shafts; and ectothrix, with the presence of fungal structures (arthroconidia and/or hyphae) within and on the exterior the hair shaft [2]. The clinical appearance of tinea capitis is variable, depending on the type of hair invasion, the level of host resistance and the degree of inflammatory host response. The pattern varies from a few, broken-off hairs with coexisted scaling, to a severe, painful, inflammatory mass or kerion covering most of the scalp. Local lymphadenopathy and itching may also occur [3]. Although mycological examination is considered to be the gold standard diagnostic method in tinea capitis, trichoscopy may be useful to establish the initial diagnosis. Characteristic trichoscopic findings of tinea capitis include comma hairs, corkscrew hairs, morse code-like hair, zigzag hairs, bent hairs, block hairs and i-hairs [1]. Examination with Wood's lamp reveals green fluorescence in the cause of *Microsporum canis* infection. Mycological examination consists of direct microscopy (with potassium hydroxide) as well as fungal culture. In the treatment of tinea capitis, systemic antifungal medications such as terbinafine, itraconazole, griseofulvin and fluconazole are recommended. Antifungal shampoos and creams may be additionally used. The treatment typically lasts four to eight weeks [4].

Differential diagnoses for the presented patient were seborrheic dermatitis, alopecia areata and psoriasis.

Seborrheic dermatitis presents as well-delineated erythematous plaques with greasy-looking, yellowish scales [5]. The scalp is most commonly affected, however the disease can also appear on the other body areas such as the face, chest, back, axilla, and groin [5, 6]. Seborrheic dermatitis is more frequently aggravated during winter and usually improves during summer [5].

Alopecia areata, a form of non-scarring autoimmune hair loss, is characterized by the presence of hair loss areas within the skin which remains normal. Although the scalp is most commonly affected, hair loss may also be observed in other hair-bearing areas (such as eyebrows, eyelashes, pubic and axillary areas). Reticular alopecia areata is characterized by a net-like pattern with multiple active and regressing patches. No scaling is observed [7].

Scalp psoriasis is characterized by the presence of red, thickened plaques with silver-white scale, either contained within the hairline, or extending onto the forehead, ears, and posterior neck. The frontal and occipital areas are most commonly affected. Itch may be reported [8].

In the presented patient, skin-scale and hair samples were collected for direct microscopic examination using the potassium hydroxide technique, which revealed hyphae. Fungal culture was positive for Trichophyton rubrum. The diagnosis of tinea capitis was established. The patient was treated with oral terbinafine at dose 250 mg daily and ketoconazole shampoo for four weeks.

Key Points
- Tinea capitis is a dermatophytosis of the scalp that most commonly affects children
- Clinical manifestation of tinea capitis varies from a few, broken-off hairs with coexisted scaling, to a severe, painful, inflammatory mass or kerion

References

1. Waskiel-Burnat A, Rakowska A, Sikora M, Ciechanowicz P, Olszewska M, Rudnicka L. Trichoscopy of tinea capitis: a systematic review. Dermatol Ther (Heidelb). 2020;10(1):43–52.
2. Peixoto RRGB, Meneses OMS, da Silva FO, Donati A, Veasey JV. Tinea capitis: correlation of clinical aspects, findings on direct mycological examination, and agents isolated from fungal culture. Int J Trichol. 2019;11(6):232–5.
3. Hay RJ. Tinea capitis: current status. Mycopathologia. 2017;182(1–2):87–93.
4. Al Aboud AM, Crane JS. Tinea capitis. StatPearls. Treasure Island (FL): StatPearls Publishing Copyright © 2020, StatPearls Publishing LLC; 2020.
5. Clark GW, Pope SM, Jaboori KA. Diagnosis and treatment of seborrheic dermatitis. Am Fam Physician. 2015;91(3):185–90.
6. Borda LJ, Wikramanayake TC. Seborrheic dermatitis and dandruff: a comprehensive review. J Clin Investig Dermatol. 2015;3(2). https://doi.org/10.13188/2373-1044.1000019.
7. Waskiel A, Rakowska A, Sikora M, Olszewska M, Rudnicka L. Trichoscopy of alopecia areata: an update. J Dermatol. 2018;45(6):692–700.
8. Blakely K, Gooderham M. Management of scalp psoriasis: current perspectives. Psoriasis (Auckl). 2016;6:33–40.

Chapter 3
A 19-Year-Old Man with Folliculitis and Hair Loss

Anna Waśkiel-Burnat, Joanna Czuwara, Małgorzata Olszewska, and Lidia Rudnicka

A 19-year-old man presented with a two-year history of recurrent folliculitis. He reported two episodes of folliculitis with single areas of hair loss during the last two years. The patient was previously treated with oral lymecycline for two–three weeks with complete resolution of skin lesions and hair regrowth. The patient did not complain of any symptoms. No history of other dermatological condition was reported.

On physical examination, widespread erythematous papules on the frontal, vertex and occipital areas were observed (Fig. 3.1). Moreover, a few small areas of non-scarring hair loss were detected. On trichoscopy black dots, yellow dots and upright regrowing hairs were presented (Fig. 3.2).

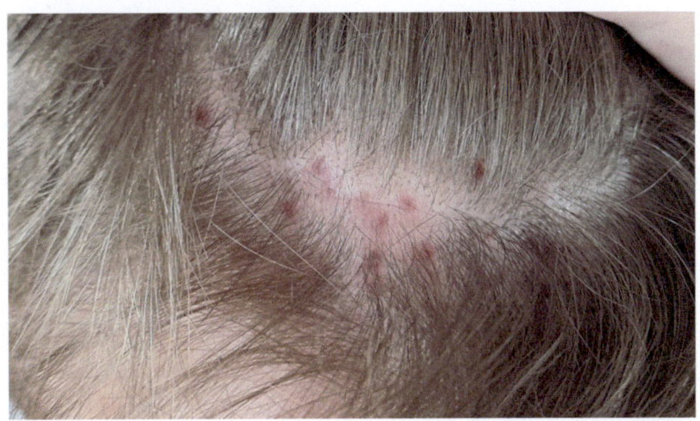

Fig. 3.1 A 19-year-old man with erythematous papules and areas of non-scarring hair loss

A. Waśkiel-Burnat (✉) · J. Czuwara · M. Olszewska · L. Rudnicka
Department of Dermatology, Medical University of Warsaw, Warsaw, Poland
e-mail: anna.waskiel@wum.edu.pl; joanna.czuwara@wum.edu.pl;
malgorzata.olszcwska@wum.edu.pl; lidia.rudnicka@wum.edu.pl

A. Waśkiel-Burnat et al. (eds.), *Clinical Cases in Hair Disorders*, Clinical Cases in Dermatology, https://doi.org/10.1007/978-3-030-93423-1_3

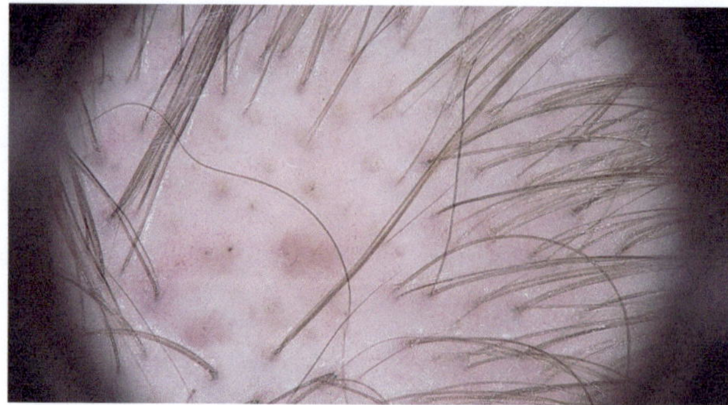

Fig. 3.2 Trichoscopy shows single black dots and yellow dots (×20)

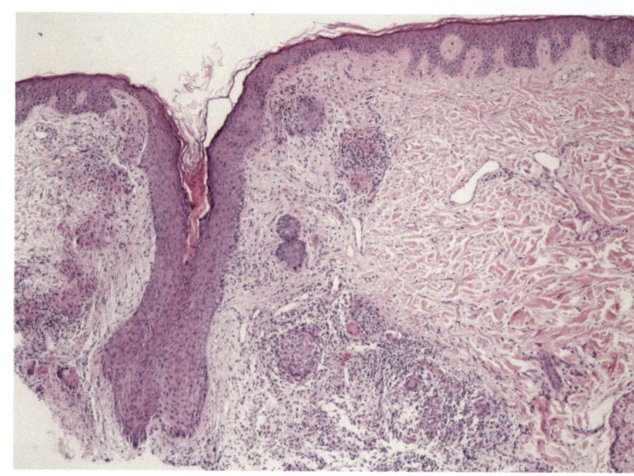

Fig. 3.3 A histopathological examination shows the mixed cell inflammatory infiltrate in the dermis extending into the subcutaneous adipose tissue. The terminal hair presents infundibular hyperkeratosis and acanthosis of the hair epithelium

A histopathological examination showed the mixed cell inflammatory infiltrate with collagen edema deeply seated in the dermis and extending into the subcutaneous adipose tissue. The terminal hair presented infundibular hyperkeratosis and acanthosis of the hair epithelium. There was a granulation tissue formation with granulomas around remnants of a damaged hairs in the deep dermis. In the upper dermis dilated blood vessels were visible (Fig. 3.3).

Based on the case description and the photographs, what is your diagnosis?

Differential Diagnoses

1. Superficial bacterial folliculitis.
2. Folliculitis decalvans.
3. Alopecia areata.
4. Early stage of dissecting cellulitis.

Diagnosis

An early stage of dissecting cellulitis.

Discussion

Dissecting cellulitis is a form of primary neutrophilic cicatricial alopecia [1]. The precise pathogenesis of dissecting cellulitis is not fully elucidated. However the role of hyperkeratosis, follicular occlusion and subsequent inflammation has been described [2]. Dissecting cellulitis most commonly affects young men of African descent. Early stage of the disease is characterized by the presence of multiple firm, violaceous papules which coalesce to form plaques and nodules. The vertex and occipital areas are most commonly affected. However, the whole scalp may be involved. The diagnosis of dissecting cellulitis is mainly based on clinical and histopathological features. Trichoscopy can be useful to avoid the scalp biopsy. At an early stage of the disease black and yellow dots predominate [3]. A histopathogical examination of an early stage of dissecting folliculitis is characterized by the presence of a lymphocytic infiltrate in the lower dermis extending into the subcutis [1]. An early diagnosis and effective treatment of dissecting cellulitis is very important because it may prevent scarring alopecia. The treatment options include topical or intralesional corticosteroids, topical antibiotics, systemic antibiotics (ciprofloxacin, clindamycin, rifampin, and trimethoprim/sulfamethaxole) and isotretinoin. Systemic corticosteroids and tumor necrosis factor inhibitors may be also useful [1].

Differential diagnoses for the presented patient included superficial bacterial folliculitis, folliculitis decalvans and alopecia areata.

Superficial bacterial folliculitis is an infection of the follicular ostium, which manifests with painful perifollicular pustular lesions with surrounding erythema. The disease is most commonly due to *Staphylococcus aureus* infection. However, *Streptococcus*, *Proteus* and *Pseudomonas* may be also causative agent. The lesions may be localized on each body area but is most often diagnosed on the scalp, beard, axilla, buttocks and extremities. No hair loss is observed [4, 5].

Folliculitis decalvans most commonly occurs in young to middle-aged men. The disease is initially characterized by follicular papules and pustules. Subsequently, tufted hairs, erosions, hemorrhagic crusts, and nodules are detected. Lesions are most commonly localized on the vertex, parietal and occipital areas. Moreover, folliculitis decalvans has been noted in other locations, including the face, neck, axillae and pubic region [1, 5].

Alopecia areata, a form of non-scarring autoimmune hair loss, is characterized by the presence of hair loss areas within the skin which remains normal. Although the scalp is most commonly affected, hair loss may also be observed in other hair-bearing areas (such as eyebrows, eyelashes, pubic and axillary areas [6]. Trichoscopic features of alopecia areata are black dots, broken hairs, exclamation mark hairs, tapered hairs, vellus hairs, yellow dots, upright regrowing hairs, pigtail (circle) hairs, and Pohl-Pinkus constrictions.

In the presented patient based on the clinical, trichoscopic and histopathological features the diagnosis of dissecting cellulitis was established. Treatment with oral isotretinoin (20 mg daily) with topical antibiotics was initiated.

Key Points
- An early stage of dissecting cellulitis is characterized by the presence of papular lesions
- At an early stage of the disease, non-scarring hair loss may be observed
- An early diagnosis and effective treatment of dissecting cellulitis may prevent scarring alopecia

References

1. Kanti V, Rowert-Huber J, Vogt A, Blume-Peytavi U. Cicatricial alopecia. J Dtsch Dermatol Ges. 2018;16(4):435–61.
2. Bolduc C, Sperling LC, Shapiro J. Primary cicatricial alopecia: other lymphocytic primary cicatricial alopecias and neutrophilic and mixed primary cicatricial alopecias. J Am Acad Dermatol. 2016;75(6):1101–17.
3. Melo DF, Lemes LR, Pirmez R, Duque-Estrada B. Trichoscopic stages of dissecting cellulitis: a potential complementary tool to clinical assessment. An Bras Dermatol. 2020;95(4):514–7.
4. Lugović-Mihić L, Barisić F, Bulat V, Buljan M, Situm M, Bradić L, et al. Differential diagnosis of the scalp hair folliculitis. Acta Clin Croat. 2011;50(3):395–402.
5. Fanti PA, Baraldi C, Misciali C, Piraccini BM. Cicatricial alopecia. G Ital Dermatol Venereol. 2018;153(2):230–42.
6. Waskiel A, Rakowska A, Sikora M, Olszewska M, Rudnicka L. Trichoscopy of alopecia areata: an update. J Dermatol. 2018;45(6):692–700.

Chapter 4
A 26-Year-Old Woman with Multiple Erythematous Areas with Coexisted Hair Loss

Anna Waśkiel-Burnat, Małgorzata Olszewska, and Lidia Rudnicka

A 26-year-old woman presented with a six-month history of multiple erythematous lesions with coexisted hair loss and itching. No history of dermatologic or non-dermatological diseases was reported.

A physical examination revealed an area of non-scarring hair loss (9 cm × 6 cm) with the central erythema on the vertex and occipital areas (Fig. 4.1). Moreover erythematous lesions with follicular keratosis and coexisted hair loss on the trunk, upper and lower extremities were presented. A histopathological examination showed a mucin deposition within the hair follicles and sebaceous glands.

Based on the case description and the photographs, what is your diagnosis?

Differential Diagnoses

1. Mycosis fungoides.
2. Alopecia areata.
3. Primary follicular mucinosis.
4. Graham-Little syndrome.

Diagnosis

Primary follicular mucinosis.

A. Waśkiel-Burnat (✉) · M. Olszewska · L. Rudnicka
Department of Dermatology, Medical University of Warsaw, Warsaw, Poland
e-mail: anna.waskiel@wum.edu.pl; malgorzata.olszewska@wum.edu.pl;
lidia.rudnicka@wum.edu.pl

A. Waśkiel-Burnat et al. (eds.), *Clinical Cases in Hair Disorders*, Clinical Cases in Dermatology, https://doi.org/10.1007/978-3-030-93423-1_4

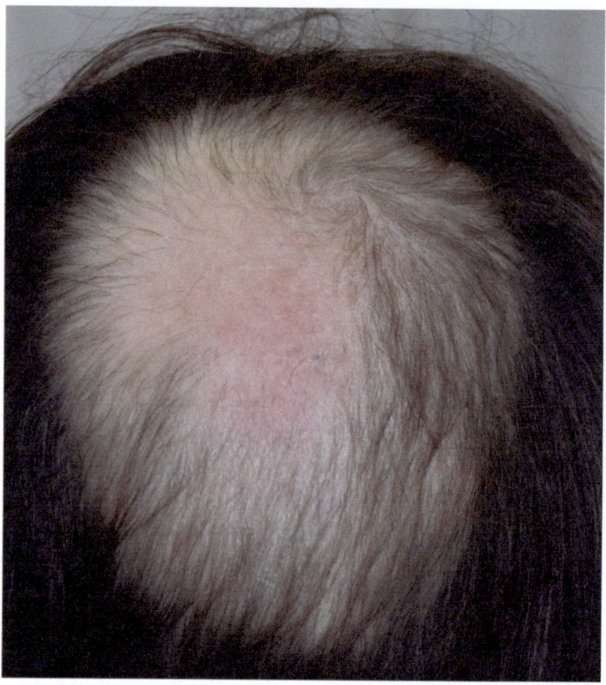

Fig. 4.1 A 26-yeard old woman with an area of non-scarring hair loss with the central erythema on the vertex and occipital areas

Discussion

Follicular mucinosis, also known as alopecia mucinosa, is a form of cutaneous mucinosis characterized by accumulation of dermal type of mucin in the pilosebaceous follicle and sebaceous glands [1]. Pathogenesis of the disease is not fully understood. There are two main clinicopathological forms of follicular mucinosis: a primary, benign variant and a secondary [1]. The primary form affects mainly children and young adults with the age range from 11 to 35 years [2]. Clinically, the disease is characterized by the presence of well-delimited, erythematous or brownish-erythematous papules, patches or plaques. Follicular keratosis or areas of alopecia may be presented. Hair loss in the course of follicular mucinosis is typically non-scarring and reversible; in very rare cases, scarring may occur [3]. The disease can be observed in any body area, however the scalp, neck and upper extremities are most commonly affected [1]. Other clinical variants of primary follicular mucinosis include the urticaria-like and acneiform. The diagnosis of follicular mucinosis is based on the clinicopathologic correlation. In histopathologic examination mucin deposits on the outer root sheath of the hair follicle, in addition to inflammatory infiltrates composed of lymphocytes, macrophages and eosinophils with folliculotropic lymphocytes are presented [4]. Mild-to-moderate potency topical corticosteroids are usually the first-line therapy for primary follicular mucinosis. Other therapeutic modalities include topical and oral antibiotics, retinoids, dapsone, imiquimod, topical pimecrolimus, and psoralen plus ultraviolet A (PUVA).

Differential diagnoses for the presented patient included mycosis fungoides, alopecia areata and Graham-Little syndrome.

Mycosis fungoides is the most common type of primary cutaneous T-cell lymphoma. It occurs more frequently in older adults and is more commonly observed in men compared to women. There are three main stages of cutaneous involvement of mucosis fungoides: patchy-, plaque, and tumor-stage. Lesions affects mainly photo-protected areas, in particular the buttocks, groin, breasts, upper thighs, and axilla and, less commonly, the distal extremities, head, and neck [4].

Alopecia areata, a form of non-scarring autoimmune hair loss, is characterized by the presence of hair loss areas within the skin which remains normal. Although the scalp is most commonly affected, hair loss can also be observed in other hair-bearing areas (such as eyebrows, eyelashes, pubic and axillary areas) [5].

Graham-Little syndrome, a variant of lichen planopilaris, is characterized by a triad consisting of patchy cicatricial alopecia of the scalp, non-cicatricial axillary and pubic hair loss and lichenoid follicular eruption. Middle-aged women are most commonly affected [3].

Based on the clinical manifestation and histopathological findings the diagnosis of primary follicular mucinosis was established. PUVA therapy and topical mometasone furoate were initiated.

Key Points
- Primary follicular mucinosis is a form of follicular mucinosis that affects mainly children and young adults
- It is characterized by the presence of well-delimited, erythematous or brownish-erythematous papules or plaques with or without alopecia

References

1. Khalil J, Kurban M, Abbas O. Follicular mucinosis: a review. Int J Dermatol. 2021;60(2):159–65. https://doi.org/10.1111/ijd.15165.
2. Alikhan A, Griffin J, Nguyen N, Davis DM, Gibson LE. Pediatric follicular mucinosis: presentation, histopathology, molecular genetics, treatment, and outcomes over an 11-year period at the Mayo Clinic. Pediatr Dermatol. 2013;30(2):192–8.
3. Kanti V, Rowert-Huber J, Vogt A, Blume-Peytavi U. Cicatricial alopecia. J Dtsch Dermatol Ges. 2018;16(4):435–61.
4. Pincus LB. Mycosis Fungoides. Surg Pathol Clin. 2014;7(2):143–67.
5. Waskiel A, Rakowska A, Sikora M, Olszewska M, Rudnicka L. Trichoscopy of alopecia areata: an update. J Dermatol. 2018;45(6):692–700.

Chapter 5
A 29-Year-Old Woman with Treatment-Resistant Dandruff

Mariusz Sikora

A 29-year-old woman presented with a two-year history of erythematous and scaly eruption on the scalp. The patient was previously treated by a general practitioner with antifungal shampoos containing ketoconazole or ciclopirox, without significant and long-term improvement. Her medical history was unremarkable. The patient denied any family history of dermatological disorders.

A physical examination of the scalp revealed erythematous plaques with overlying whitish scales extending onto the forehead (Fig. 5.1). No other skin, mucosal or

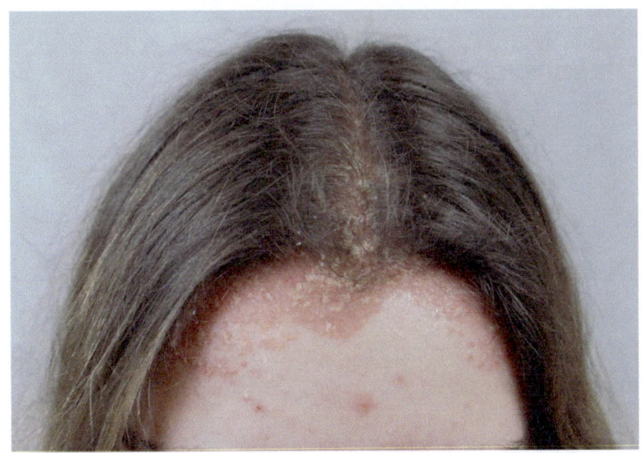

Fig. 5.1 A 29-year-old woman with erythematous and scaly eruptions on the scalp

M. Sikora (✉)
National Institute of Geriatrics, Rheumatology and Rehabilitation, Warsaw, Poland
e-mail: mariusz.sikora@spartanska.pl

© The Author(s), under exclusive license to Springer Nature Switzerland AG 2022
A. Waśkiel-Burnat et al. (eds.), *Clinical Cases in Hair Disorders*, Clinical Cases in Dermatology, https://doi.org/10.1007/978-3-030-93423-1_5

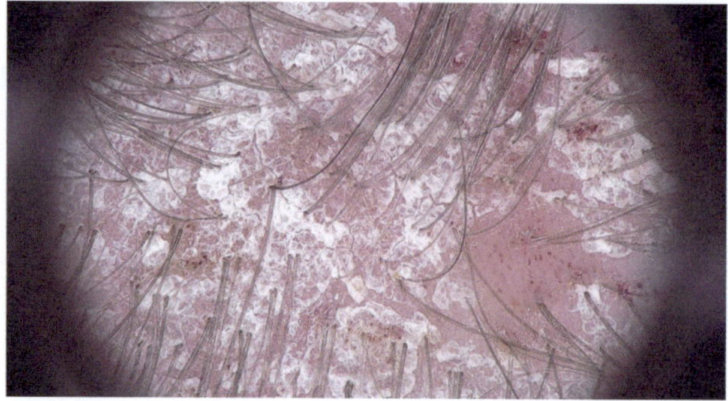

Fig. 5.2 Trichoscopy shows red dots, twisted capillary loops, punctate hemorrhages and white scales (×20)

nail changes were presented. Trichoscopy showed red dots, twisted capillary loops, punctate hemorrhages and white scales (Fig. 5.2).

Based on the case description and the photographs, what is your diagnosis?

Differential Diagnoses

1. Tinea capitis.
2. Seborrheic dermatitis.
3. Scalp psoriasis.
4. Allergic contact dermatitis.

Diagnosis

Scalp psoriasis.

Discussion

Psoriasis is a chronic, systemic inflammatory skin disease that affects approximately 1–3% of the world population. The exact etiology is unknown, but psoriasis is considered to be an autoimmune, genetically predisposed disease mediated by T lymphocytes. The disease may present at any age with bimodal age of onset. The mean age of onset for the first presentation of psoriasis ranges from 15 to 20 years of age, with a second peak occurring at 55 to 60 years. The disease is characterized by the presence of erythematous papules and plaques covered with silvery scales. Morphologically it is classified as plaque, guttate, rupioid, erythrodermic, pustular, inverse, and elephantine. Site variation is observed with the involvement of the scalp, palmoplantar region, genitals, and nails [1, 2].

Scalp psoriasis is one of the most common form of plaque psoriasis, with up to 80% of patients experiencing scalp involvement at some time point of the disease. Scalp lesions can be the first manifestation of psoriasis and persist for many years. It is also suggested that the presence of scalp psoriasis is a possible prognostic marker for the future development of psoriatic arthritis [1, 2]. The characteristic lesions of scalp psoriasis consist of sharply demarcated erythematous plaques with silvery-white scales, which may extend beyond the hairline. Scalp psoriasis affects several dimensions of patients' quality of life irrespective of disease severity in other areas of the body. The visibility of the lesions and scaling causes low self-esteem with a great impact on social activity. Pruritus is one of the most frequent and distressing symptoms in scalp psoriasis impacting the quality of life. Hair loss associated with scalp psoriasis can add to the already substantial burden of the disease [3, 4].

The diagnosis of psoriasis in mainly established based on clinical manifestation. Dermoscopy may be helpful to confirm the initial diagnosis. In scalp psoriasis, trichoscopy shows red dots at a low magnification and twisted/glomerular capillary loops at a higher magnification. Additional features include red loops, hairpin vessels, white scales, and punctate hemorrhages [5]. In ambigous cases, especially in skin lesions limited to the scalp area, skin biopsy with histopathological examination is suggested. Histopathological findings of psoriasis are epidermal acanthosis (thickening of viable layers), hyperkeratosis (thickened cornified layer), and parakeratosis (cell nuclei present in the cornified layer) [1–3].

Scalp psoriasis often requires different treatment strategies from those used on other body areas, remaining one of the most difficult-to-manage forms of the disease. This is partly due to the high density of hair follicles and pilosebaceous units which make difficulties in reaching the scalp surface for topical treatments or phototherapy. Furthermore, several formulations of topical products are poorly accepted by the patients due to unpleasant cosmetic effects, often leading to poor patient satisfaction and compliance [6–8]. Topical agents are considered as the first-line therapeutic option. The combination of calcipotriene and betamethasone dipropionate is most commonly used. Other topical therapies include topical or intralesional corticosteroids, retinoids, anthralin, tar and keratolytic agents [6–8]. Recalcitrant or more severe disease may require systemic treatment. However, effectiveness of conventional oral systemic agents, such as methotrexate, acitretin and cyclosporine, have been studied in the treatment of generalized psoriasis. The data regarding their efficacy and safety in scalp psoriasis, are based on low-quality evidence. The effectiveness of biologics and small molecules (apremilast) in scalp psoriasis has been confirmed in a higher number of clinical trials. Most of available evidence has been obtained by the sub-analysis of trials in which scalp involvement was additionally assessed. Etanercept, secukinumab and apremilast determined the efficacy in scalp psoriasis in predefined studies [8].

Differential diagnosis of scalp psoriasis can be challenging due to similar clinical features of diseases that involve the scalp and their possible overlapping [9, 10]. Differential diasnoses for the presented patient included tinea capitis, seborrheic dermatitis and allergic contact dermatitis.

Tinea capitis, a fungal infection of the scalp, affects mainly children. The disease is characterized by the presence of hair loss areas with coexisted scaling, inflammation or pustules.

Seborrheic dermatitis is a chronic inflammatory dermatological condition. It presents as well-demarkated erythematous plaques with greasy-looking, yellowish scales. The scalp is most commonly affected; however, the disease can appear also on the other body areas such as the face, chest, back, axilla, and groin. Seborrheic dermatitis is characterized by a seasonal pattern, presenting more frequently during winter, and improving usually during summer [4].

Allergic contact dermatitis is an inflammatory eczematous skin disease. The disease is rarely presented on the scalp area because of the great thickness of the epidermis in this region. In the case of application of irritants or allergens on the scalp symptoms are usually observed on the face or neck area. Clinically, contact dermatitis presents as an erythema with scaling and coexisting itch. In acute disease, vesicles or pustules may be present [5].

In the presented patient, based on the clinical and dermoscopic features, the diagnosis of scalp psoriasis was established. The treatment with calcipotriene 0.005% and betamethasone dipropionate 0.064% gel was initiated.

Key Points
- Scalp psoriasis is prevalent and difficult to treat disease that has negative impact on patients' quality of life
- It present as sharply demarcated erythematous plaques with silvery-white scales, which may extend beyond the hairline
- While topical therapies are considered the first-line therapeutic option, recalcitrant scalp psoriasis may require systemic agents

References

1. Nair PA, Badri T. Psoriasis. StatPearls. Treasure Island (FL): StatPearls Publishing Copyright © 2020, StatPearls Publishing LLC; 2020.
2. Dopytalska K, Sobolewski P, Błaszczak A, Szymańska E, Walecka I. Psoriasis in special localizations. Reumatologia. 2018;56(6):392–8.
3. Lanna C, Galluzzi C, Zangrilli A, Bavetta M, Bianchi L, Campione E. Psoriasis in difficult to treat areas: treatment role in improving health-related quality of life and perception of the disease stigma. J Dermatolog Treat. 2020;28:1–4.
4. Golińska J, Sar-Pomian M, Rudnicka L. Dermoscopic features of psoriasis of the skin, scalp and nails - a systematic review. J Eur Acad Dermatol Venereol. 2019;33(4):648–60.
5. Widaty S, Pusponegoro EH, Rahmayunita G, Astriningrum R, Akhmad AM, Oktarina C, Miranda E, Agustin T. Applicability of Trichoscopy in scalp seborrheic dermatitis. Int J Trichol. 2019;11(2):43–8.

6. Chan CS, Van Voorhees AS, Lebwohl MG, Korman NJ, Young M, Bebo BF Jr, Kalb RE, Hsu S. Treatment of severe scalp psoriasis: from the medical Board of the National Psoriasis Foundation. J Am Acad Dermatol. 2009;60(6):962–71.
7. Ortonne J, Chimenti S, Luger T, Puig L, Reid F, Trüeb RM. Scalp psoriasis: European consensus on grading and treatment algorithm. J Eur Acad Dermatol Venereol. 2009;23(12): 1435–44.
8. Reich A, Adamski Z, Chodorowska G, Kaszuba A, Krasowska D, Lesiak A, Maj J, Narbutt J, Osmola-Mańkowska A, Owczarczyk-Saczonek A, Owczarek W, Placek W, Rudnicka L, Szepietowski J. Psoriasis. Diagnostic and therapeutic recommendations of the Polish Dermatological Society. Part 1. Dermatology Review/Przegląd Dermatologiczny. 2020;107(2):92–108.
9. Clark GW, Pope SM, Jaboori KA. Diagnosis and treatment of seborrheic dermatitis. Am Fam Physician. 2015;91(3):185–90.
10. Rozas-Muñoz E, Gamé D, Serra-Baldrich E. Allergic contact dermatitis by anatomical regions: diagnostic clues. Actas Dermosifiliogr. 2018;109(6):485–507.

Chapter 6
A 34-Year-Old Man with an Indurated Alopecic Lesion on the Scalp

Mateusz Kamiński, Anna Waśkiel-Burnat, Mariusz Sikora, and Magdalena Jasińska

A 36-year-old man presented with a five-year history of multiple indurated lesions localized on the scalp, face, trunk and extremities. Initially, the lesions involved the upper extremities followed by the trunk, face and scalp. He complained of mild itch and denied having other symptoms. The patient had epilepsy and scoliosis.

A physical examination revealed shiny area of scarring hair loss with the presence of arborizing vessels on the left side of the frontoparietal area. Non scarring hair loss was presented on the vertex and frontotemporal regions (Fig. 6.1). Moreover, multiple, polycyclic, indurated, pigmented plaques with solitary white

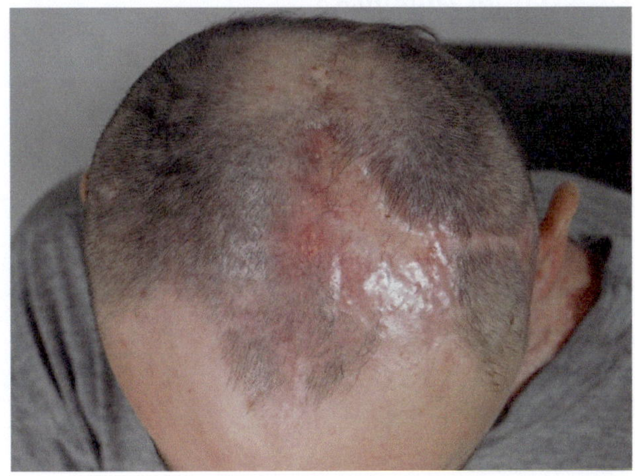

Fig. 6.1 A 34-year-old with the presence of shiny area of scarring hair loss with arborizing vessels on left side of the frontoparietal area. Non scarring hair loss on the vertex and frontotemporal regions is also observed

M. Kamiński (✉) · A. Waśkiel-Burnat · M. Sikora · M. Jasińska
Department of Dermatology, Medical University of Warsaw, Warsaw, Poland
e-mail: anna.waskiel@wum.edu.pl; mariusz.sikora@wum.edu.pl

© The Author(s), under exclusive license to Springer Nature Switzerland AG 2022
A. Waśkiel-Burnat et al. (eds.), *Clinical Cases in Hair Disorders*, Clinical Cases in Dermatology, https://doi.org/10.1007/978-3-030-93423-1_6

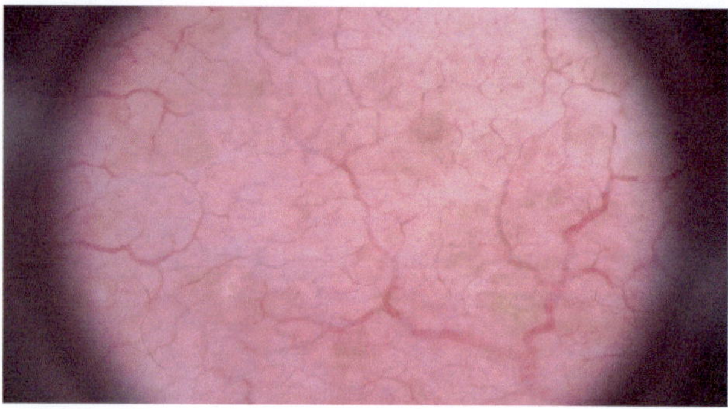

Fig. 6.2 Trichoscopy shows arborizing vessels on the erythematous background, yellowish patches and yellowish-white keratotic follicular plugs (×20)

papules were observed on the face, trunk and upper and lower extremities. No genital lesions were presented. On trichoscopy, arborizing vessels on the erythematous background, yellowish patches and yellowish-white keratotic follicular plugs and white areas with the absence of follicular openings were detected (Fig. 6.2).

A histopathological examination of the trunk lesion revealed atrophic epidermis with overlying hyperkeratosis, follicular hyperkeratosis and a band of dermal hyalinization. In the dermis below hyalinized collagen, lymphocytic dispersed band of inflammation was observed.

Based on the case description and the photographs, what is your diagnosis?

Differential Diagnoses

1. Lichen sclerosus.
2. Discoid lupus erythematosus.
3. Localized scleroderma (morphea).
4. Alopecia neoplastica.

Diagnosis

Lichen sclerosus.

Discussion

Lichen sclerosus is a chronic inflammatory disorder. The pathogenesis of the disease is not fully elucidated. However, an autoimmune etiology, genetic predisposition and the role of hormones, trauma and chronic irritation is suggested [1]. Lichen sclerosus more commonly affects women compared to men. The condition may occur at all ages. However, it is most commonly presented in prepubertal girls and postmenopausal women. Men are most commonly affected in their fourth decade of life [2]. Lichen sclerosus occurs in the genital skin in 85% to 98% of cases. The extragenital lesions are observed in 15–20% of patients and most commonly affect the inframammary areas, neck, wrists, thighs, upper back, and shoulders. The scalp involvement is rare. Typical lesions begin as a sharply demarcated erythema that becomes thin, hypopigmented, ivory-white, porcelain-like, and sclerotic plaques [3]. Plaques may become thickened due to repeated excoriations. Telangiectasias, purpura, fissures, ulcerations, and edema may be also presented. The extragenital lesions are usually asymptomatic. However, pruritus, local burning sensation and pain may occur [3]. The diagnosis of lichen sclerosus is commonly established clinically. Dermoscopy and histopathology are useful to confirm diagnosis. The most characteristic dermoscopic features of lichen sclerosus are bright white/white-yellowish patches and yellowish-white keratotic follicular plugs [4]. Specific histopathological feature of lichen sclerosus is a band-like lymphocytic infiltrate below a zone of dermal edema and orthokeratotic hyperkeratosis. At earlier stages, vacuolar degeneration of the basal layer, hyalinization of subepithelial collagen, decreased elastic fibers in the upper dermis and dilated blood vessels under the basement membrane are observed. In older lesions, a reduced number of mononuclear cells and dispersed patchy islands of mononuclear cells within the hyalinized dermis are detected [3]. Potent or ultrapotent topical corticosteroids and topical tacrolimus are usually the first-line treatment in extragenital lichen sclerosis. In more severe cases, phototherapy, systemic corticosteroids or methotrexate are recommended.

Differential diagnoses for the presented patient included morphea, discoid lupus erythematosus and basal cell carcinoma.

Discoid lupus erythematosus, a variant of chronic cutaneous lupus erythematosus, is a of lymphocytic primary cicatricial alopecia. Typically, it occurs in women between 20 and 40 years of age. The disease is characterized by circumscribed erythematous indurated plaques with coexisted scaling. When the adherent scale is removed, follicular plugging may be observed (carpet tack sign). Telangiectasias, atrophy, depigmentation, and hyperpigmentation may be detected [5].

Morphea, also known as localized scleroderma, is a rare inflammatory disease of the skin and subcutaneous tissue. Circumscribed morphea is the most common variant that is characterized by isolated oval or round lesions localized most commonly on the trunk or chest. The scalp involvement is rarely observed. Early lesions of morphea present as erythema and induration with some itching and tenderness. Later, sclerotic centres surrounded by a violaceous border are observed. The lesions result in hyperpigmentation or hypopigmentation with atrophy of the skin and subcutaneous tissue [6].

Alopecia neoplastica is a pattern of scalp metastasis. It presents as a hairless patch or a plaque with or without scaling. Subcutaneous nodule and telangiectasias may be observed [3].

In the presented patient, based on the clinical presentation, trichoscopic and histopathological findings lichen sclerosus was diagnosed. Moreover, the diagnosis of androgenetic alopecia was established. The patient was initially treated with subcutaneous methotrexate (15 mg weekly) and systemic corticosteroids (prednisone 20 mg daily) for six months without significant improvement. Cyclosporine (3 mg/kg/day) was initiated with no disease progression. The patient refused androgenetic alopecia treatment.

Key Points
- Lichen sclerosus is a chronic inflammatory condition that rarely affects the scalp area
- The disease is characterized by a sharply demarcated erythema that becomes thin, hypopigmented, ivory-white, porcelain-like, and sclerotic plaques

References

1. Kirtschig G. Lichen Sclerosus-presentation, diagnosis and management. Dtsch Arztebl Int. 2016;113(19):337–43.
2. Fistarol SK, Itin PH. Diagnosis and treatment of lichen sclerosus: an update. Am J Clin Dermatol. 2013;14(1):27–47.
3. Chamli A, Souissi A. Lichen Sclerosus. StatPearls. Treasure Island (FL): StatPearls Publishing Copyright © 2020, StatPearls Publishing LLC; 2020.
4. Errichetti E, Lallas A, Apalla Z, Di Stefani A, Stinco G. Dermoscopy of Morphea and cutaneous lichen Sclerosus: Clinicopathological correlation study and comparative analysis. Dermatology. 2017;233(6):462–70.
5. Fanti PA, Baraldi C, Misciali C, Piraccini BM. Cicatricial alopecia. G Ital Dermatol Venereol. 2018;153(2):230–42.
6. Kreuter A, Wischnewski J, Terras S, Altmeyer P, Stücker M, Gambichler T. Coexistence of lichen sclerosus and morphea: a retrospective analysis of 472 patients with localized scleroderma from a German tertiary referral center. J Am Acad Dermatol. 2012;67(6):1157–62.

Chapter 7
A 38-Year-Old Woman with Linear Hair Loss

Anna Waśkiel-Burnat, Ewelina Ulc, Małgorzata Olszewska, and Lidia Rudnicka

A 38-year-old woman presented with a two-year history of linear hair loss on the left side of the frontoparietal area of the scalp. Initially, an erythematous macula on the left side of the forehead, followed by a formation of a hypopigmented atrophic scar extending to the fronto-parietal area of the scalp was reported. The patient denied having any symptoms or traumatic injury. Non-dermatological or non-dermatological diseases were reported.

On physical examination, a 9-cm linear, alopecic plaque extending from the left side of the forehead to the frontoparietal area of the scalp was detected (Fig. 7.1).

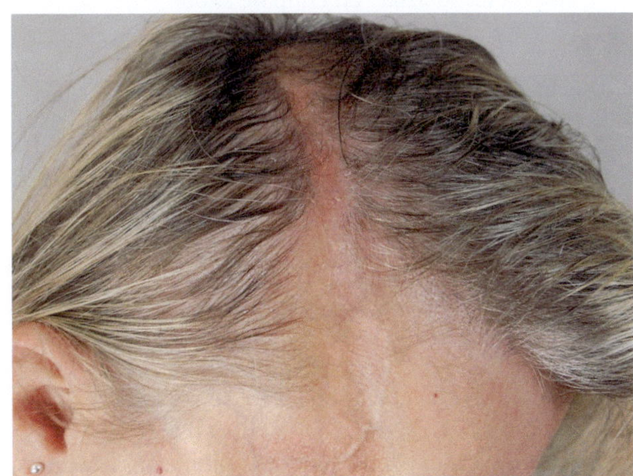

Fig. 7.1 A 38-year-old woman with linear, alopecic plaque extending from the left side of the forehead to the frontoparietal area of the scalp

A. Waśkiel-Burnat (✉) · E. Ulc · M. Olszewska · L. Rudnicka
Department of Dermatology, Medical University of Warsaw, Warsaw, Poland
e-mail: anna.waskiel@wum.edu.pl; malgorzata.olszewska@wum.edu.pl;
lidia.rudnicka@wum.edu.pl

A. Waśkiel-Burnat et al. (eds.), *Clinical Cases in Hair Disorders*, Clinical Cases in Dermatology, https://doi.org/10.1007/978-3-030-93423-1_7

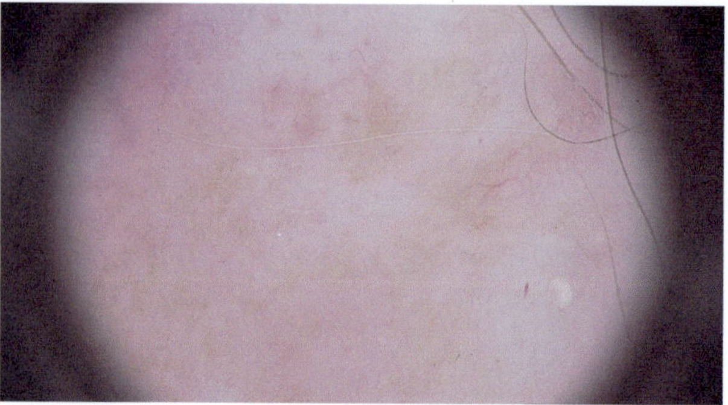

Fig. 7.2 Trichoscopy with the presence of whitish area with lack of follicular openings, honeycomb pattern and thin arborizing vessels (×20)

On trichoscopy, whitish area with lack of follicular openings, honeycomb pattern and thin arborizing vessels were observed (Fig. 7.2).

Based on the case description and the photographs, what is your diagnosis?

Differential Diagnoses

1. Linear discoid lupus erythematosus.
2. Linear lichen sclerosus.
3. Traumatic injury.
4. Linear scleroderma "en coup de sabre".

Diagnosis

Linear scleroderma "en coup de sabre".

Discussion

Linear scleroderma "en coup de sabre" is a form of linear morphea. The pathogenesis of the disease is not fully elucidated although there is increasing evidence of an autoimmune origin [1]. Environmental triggers, such as previous local trauma, have been suggested. Linear scleroderma "en coup de sabre" predominantly affects children and women and usually presents within the first two decades of life [1]. Clinically, at the early phase lesions appear as a single erythematous or violaceous linear indurated plaque with subsequent progression to hypopigmented or depigmented sclerotic deep furrow. The lesion is located on the forehead and frontoparietal area and resembles a stroke from a sabre [1]. Linear scleroderma "en coup de sabre" may be associated with a number of neurological symptoms which include headache, epilepsy, focal neurologic deficits, movement disorders, neuropsychiatric symptoms, and intellectual deterioration [2]. The diagnosis of the diseases is established clinically and confirmed on histopathological examination. Histopathologic findings of linear scleroderma 'en coup de sabre' include moderate interface dermatitis and lymphocytic infiltrate accompanied by spongiosis and dermal fibrosis [1]. On trichoscopy, whitish areas with the absence of follicular openings, scattered black dots, broken hairs, and pili torti are observed. Moreover, short thick linear and branching tortuous vessels on the periphery of the lesion are detected [3]. In 46–63% of patients with linear scleroderma "en coup de sabre", positive anti-nuclear antibodies are presented [1]. Methotrexate in monotherapy or combined with systemic corticosteroids is considered as the first-line therapeutic option. Mycophenolate mofetil, cyclosporine, and biologics therapies (abatacept, tocilizumab, interferon gamma) may be recommended for refractory linear scleroderma en coup de sabre. Additionaly, topical corticosteroids or calcineurin inhibitors may be used.

Differential diagnoses for the presented patient included linear discoid lupus erythematosus, linear lichen sclerosus and traumatic injury.

Linear discoid lupus erythematosus is a rare form of cutaneous lupus that mainly occurs in children and young adults with no gender predilection. The condition presents as single or multiple linear asymptomatic erythematous plaques along the Blashko lines. The head and neck are most commonly affected. In patients with linear discoid lupus erythematosus, the antinuclear antibodies are mostly negative [4].

Lichen sclerosus is an inflammatory dermatosis of an unclear pathogenesis, that usually affects perimenopausal and postmenopausal women. The lesions are typically localized on the vulvar, perineal and perianal area. Less commonly the palms, soles, scalp and face are affected. Linear lichen sclerosus along the Blaschko lines have been described in the literature [5].

Based on clinical manifestation and trichoscopy, diagnosis of linear scleroderma "en coup de sabre" was established. Methotrexate subcutaneous injections (15 mg once weekly) and topical tacrolimus 0.1% ointment were initiated. No disease progression was observed.

Key Points
- Linear scleroderma "en coup de sabre" is a cause of unilateral hair loss
- It presents as single erythematous or violaceous linear indurated plaque with subsequent progression to hypopigmented or depigmented sclerotic deep furrow
- The lesion is typically located on the forehead and frontoparietal area

References

1. Rattanakaemakorn P, Jorizzo JL. The efficacy of methotrexate in the treatment of en coup de sabre (linear morphea subtype). J Dermatolog Treat. 2018;29(2):197–9.
2. Arif T, Adil M, Amin SS, Sami M, Raj D. Twardzina "en coup de sabre" i twardzina ograniczona plackowata: rzadkie współistnienie. Przegląd Dermatologiczny. 2017;104(5):570–4.
3. Saceda-Corralo D, Tosti A. Trichoscopic features of linear Morphea on the scalp. Skin Appendage Disord. 2018;4(1):31–3.
4. Sindhusen S, Chanprapaph K, Rutnin S. Adult-onset linear discoid lupus erythematosus on the forehead mimicking en coup de sabre: a case report. J Med Case Rep. 2019;13(1):350.
5. Kim CR, Jung KD, Kim H, Jung M, Byun JY, Lee D-Y, et al. Linear lichen Sclerosus along the Blaschko's line of the face. Ann Dermatol. 2011;23(2):222–4.

Chapter 8
A 40-Year-Old Woman of African Descent with the Central Scalp Hair Loss

Nkechi Anne Enechukwu

A 40-year-old woman presented with a six-year history of progressive scalp hair loss. Hair loss was preceded by mild itching and no hair regrowth in the involved area. She reported hair grooming including frequent use of hot combs and application of hair dyes and chemical hair relaxers (every two months) with occasional burns. There was a history of similar pattern of hair loss in her mother. No personal or family history of diabetes mellitus, uterine leiomyoma or keloid formation was reported.

A physical examination revealed an area of scarring hair loss with the presence of papules on the vertex, parietal and frontal scalp (Fig. 8.1). The other body hair were unaffected. On trichoscopic examination, honeycomb pattern with fibrotic white patches, asterisk-like brown blotches, and white peripilar halo were observed. Additionally, there was the predominance of single-hair follicular units and perifollicular scaling (Fig. 8.2).

Based on the case description and the photographs, what is your diagnosis?

Differential Diagnoses

1. Central Centrifugal Cicatricial alopecia.
2. Alopecia areata (sisaipho pattern).
3. Lichen planopilaris.
4. Discoid lupus erythematosus.

N. A. Enechukwu (✉)
Dermatology Unit, Department of Internal Medicine, Faculty of Medicine, Nnamdi Azikiwe University, Nnewi Campus, Anambra State, Nigeria
e-mail: na.enechukwu@unizik.edu.ng

A. Waśkiel-Burnat et al. (eds.), *Clinical Cases in Hair Disorders*, Clinical Cases in Dermatology, https://doi.org/10.1007/978-3-030-93423-1_8

Fig. 8.1 A 40-year-old woman with scarring hair loss with the presence of papules on the vertex, parietal and frontal scalp

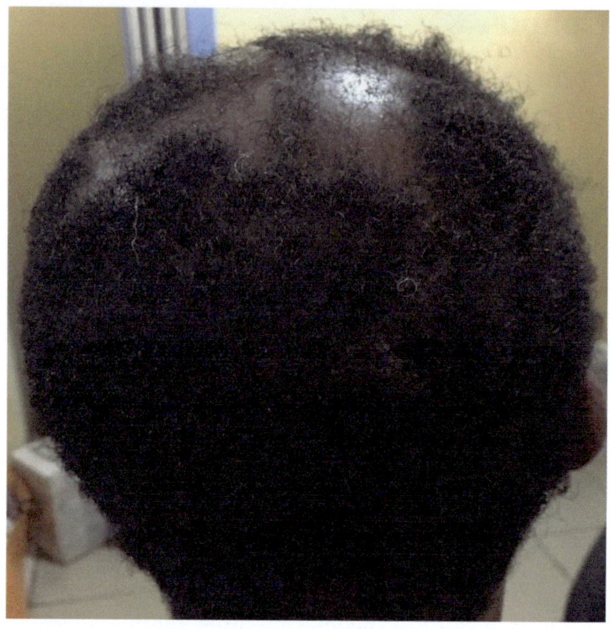

Fig. 8.2 Trichoscopy shows honeycomb pattern with fibrotic white patches, asterisk-like brown blotches, and white peripilar halo. There is a predominance of single-hair follicular units and perifollicular scaling (×20)

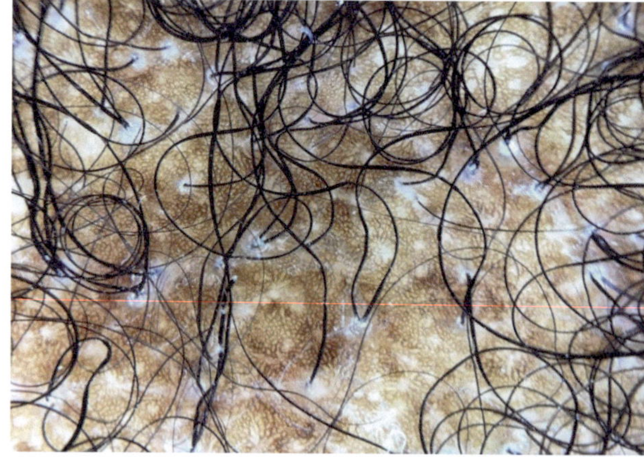

Diagnosis

Central Centrifugal Cicatricial Alopecia.

Discussion

Central centrifugal cicatricial alopecia (CCCA) is a primary lymphocytic form of scarring hair loss. The term comprises the conditions formerly referred to "hot comb alopecia", the follicular degeneration syndrome, and the pseudopelade in African Americans [1]. A multifactorial etiology is suspected. The role of various factors such as chemical straighteners, hair dyes, traction hairstyles, and bacterial or fungal infections of the scalp has been suggested [1]. Genetic predisposition with mutations in peptidyl arginine deiminase type IIII (*PADI3)* gene (an enzyme with an important role in normal hair shaft formation) have also been documented [2, 3]. Furthermore, a link between CCCA and uterine leiyomyoma, type 2 diabetes mellitus and fibrosing conditions like keloids was described [4]. The disease predominantly occurs in middle-aged women of African descent [1]. Clinically, it presents as scarring hair loss starting from the vertex area and progressively expanding in a centrifugal manner to other scalp regions. Perifollicular hyperpigmentation, erythema and islands of unaffected skin within the affected area may be detected. Itching, pain and burning sensation are frequently reported [1]. Diagnosis of CCCA is established based on clinical and histopathological correlation. Trichoscopy can be helpful to avoid the scalp biopsy. Trichoscopic features of CCCA include honeycomb pattern, asterisk-like brown blotches, white patches, peripilar white halo, paripilar dark halo, perifollicular erythema, scaling and pin point white dots [5]. Histopathological findings include premature desquamation of the inner root sheath, perifollicular lamellar fibrosis and predominantly lymphocytic, perifollicular inflammation [1]. Treatment of CCCA usually consists of potent topical and/or intralesional corticosteroids. Other therapeutic options include topical or systemic antibiotics (eg. doxycycline), oral corticosteroids, hydroxychloroquine, mycophenolate mofetil cyclosporine and minoxidil. Avoidance of chemical straighteners, hair dyes and traction inducing hairstyles is recommended [1].

The differential diagnoses for the presented patient included alopecia areata, lichen planopilaris and discoid lupus erythematosus.

Alopecia areata is an autoimmune form of non-scarring hair loss, that can affect any hair-bearing area. The disease is characterized by the presence of hairless patches within the skin that remains normal. Clinically, various patterns of alopecia areata are distinguished. Alopecia areata sisaipho is characterized by hair loss on the vertex and parietal areas sparing the temporal and occipital areas. This gives the central scalp hair loss pattern resembling CCCA. However, trichoscopy shows broken hairs, exclamation mark hairs and regrowing hairs. Perifollicular fibrosis is rarely observed in alopecia areata and it is limited to the long-lasting cases [6].

Lichen planopilaris is a primary lymphocytic form of scarring alopecia. Caucasians aged 40–60 years are most commonly affected. Women are more frequently affected than men [1]. Lichen planopilaris presents as cicatricial hair loss areas with the presence of perifollicular erythema and follicular hyperkeratosis at the periphery that predominantly affects the vertex and parietal area [3].

Discoid lupus erythematosus, a variant of chronic cutaneous lupus erythematosus, is a form of lymphocytic primary cicatricial alopecia. Typically, it occurs in women between 20 and 40 years of age. The condition is more commonly diagnosed in African-Americans compared to Caucasians [1]. The disease is characterized by circumscribed erythematous indurated plaques with coexisted scaling. When the adherent scale is removed, follicular plugging may be observed (carpet tack sign). Telangiectasias, dilated plugged follicles, atrophy, depigmentation, and hyperpigmentation may be detected [7].

In the presented patient, based on the clinical presentation and trichoscopic findings, the diagnosis of CCCA was established. She was treated with oral doxycycline, intralesional triamcinolone acetonide and topical minoxidil. The avoidance of traction inducing hairstyles, hot combs and chemical hair relaxers for hair grooming was also recommended.

Key Points
- Central centrifugal cicatricial alopecia (CCCA) is a common cause of cicatricial alopecia in women of African descent
- It presents as scarring hair loss starting from the vertex area and progressively expanding in a centrifugal manner to other scalp regions

References

1. Kanti V, Rowert-Huber J, Vogt A, Blume-Peytavi U. Cicatricial alopecia. J Dtsch Dermatol Ges. 2018;16(4):435–61.
2. Dlova NC, Jordaan FH, Sarig O, Sprecher E. Autosomal dominant inheritance of central centrifugal cicatricial alopecia in black south Africans. J Am Acad Dermatol. 2014;70(4):679–82.e1.
3. Malki L, Sarig O, Romano MT, Méchin MC, Peled A, Pavlovsky M, et al. Variant PADI3 in central centrifugal cicatricial Alopecia. N Engl J Med. 2019;380(9):833–41.
4. Whiting DA. Cicatricial alopecia: clinico-pathological findings and treatment. Clin Dermatol. 2001;19(2):211–25.
5. Mathur M, Acharya P. Trichoscopy of primary cicatricial alopecias: an updated review. J Eur Acad Dermatol Venereol. 2020;34(3):473–84. https://doi.org/10.1111/jdv.15974.
6. Whiting DA. Histopathologic features of alopecia areata: a new look. Arch Dermatol. 2003;139(12):1555–9.
7. Fanti PA, Baraldi C, Misciali C, Piraccini BM. Cicatricial alopecia. G Ital Dermatol Venereol. 2018;153(2):230–42.

Chapter 9
A 52-Year-Old Woman with Scarring Alopecia

Justyna Milewska and Agnieszka Gradzińska

A 52-year-old woman was presented with a ten-year history of alopecia, gradually evolving over the last several months. The scalp lesions were associated with intermittent itching. There was no personal history of dermatological or non-dermatological diseases.

On the physical examination, four erythematous plaques with scaling and atrophic areas on the frontal, left retroauricular and parietal regions were presented (Fig. 9.1). Trichoscopy showed arborizing vessels, diffuse whitish scaling and whitish areas lacking of follicular openings (Fig. 9.2).

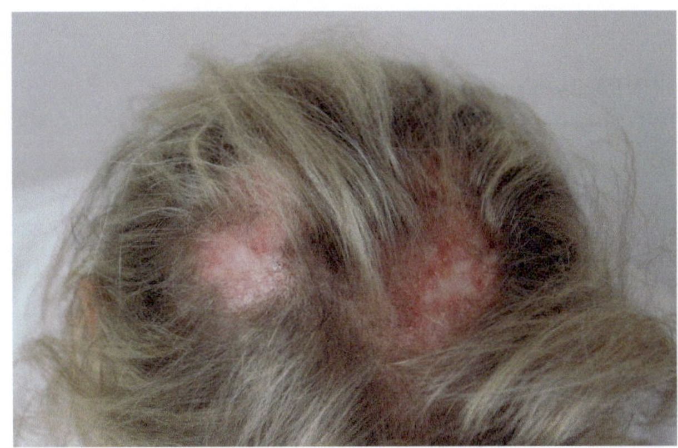

Fig. 9.1 A 52-year-old woman with erythematous plaques with scaling and atrophic areas on the parietal area

J. Milewska (✉) · A. Gradzińska
Department of Dermatology, Medical University of Warsaw, Warsaw, Poland

A. Waśkiel-Burnat et al. (eds.), *Clinical Cases in Hair Disorders*, Clinical Cases in Dermatology, https://doi.org/10.1007/978-3-030-93423-1_9

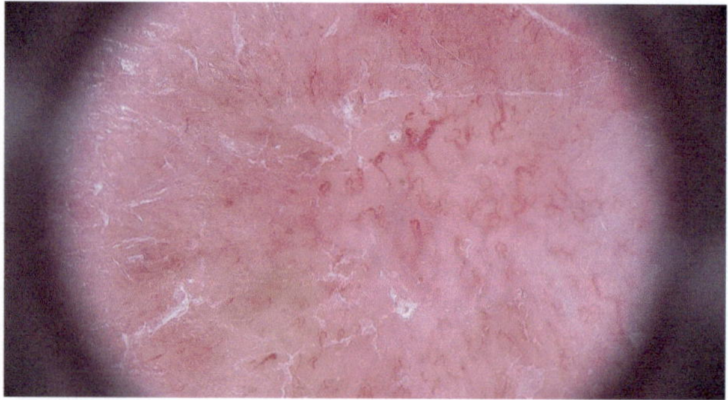

Fig. 9.2 Trichoscopy shows arborizing vessels and diffuse, whitish scaling (×20)

Laboratory tests were normal. Antinuclear antibodies were not detected. In histopathology, follicular hyperkeratosis with a dense, partially perifollicular infiltrate of lymphocytes and histiocytes were observed.

Based on the case description and the photographs, what is your diagnosis?

Differential Diagnoses

1. Lichen planopilaris.
2. Pseudopelade of Brocq.
3. Discoid lupus erythematosus.
4. Brunsting-Perry cicatricial pemphigoid.

Diagnosis

Discoid lupus erythematosus.

Discussion

Discoid lupus erythematosus is a chronic, photosensitive, scarring dermatosis. It is considered being one of the most frequent primary lymphocytic scarring alopecia [1]. It affects mainly women, between 20–40 years of age [2]. The disease may occur in patients with systemic lupus erythematosus. However, systemic lupus erythematous is diagnosed in only 5–10% of patients with discoid lupus erythematous [3]. Discoid lupus erythematous initially presents as round or discoid, well-circumscribed, erythematosus plaques with adherent follicular hyperkeratosis. Hyperpigmentation may be also observed [1, 3, 4]. Unlike other cicatricial alopecias, telangiectasia and scale are usually more prominent on the center of the alopecic plaques [4]. Tenderness or pruritus may occur. Early lesions of discoid lupus erythematosus may be only slightly inflammatory and non-scarring. Later, they progress toward a sclero-atrophic, white-ivory plaques [1]. The scalp area is most commonly affected [4]. The diagnosis of discoid lupus erythematosus is established based on clinical picture, immunofluorescence tests and histopathological examination. Trichoscopy can be helpful to avoid the scalp biopsy [5]. Characteristic trichoscopic findings of discoid lupus erythematosus include large yellow dots, red dots and large yellow dots with radial, thin arborizing vessels emerging from the dot (also known as "red spider in yellow dot"). Other typical trichoscopic features of the disease are thick arborizing vessels, scattered dark-brown discoloration and blue-grey dots arranged in a "speckled" pattern. The most characteristic histopathological features of discoid lupus erythematosus are an interface dermatitis, lymphohistiocytic infiltration around the vessels and appendages, follicular keratotic plugs, mucin deposition, and basement membrane thickening [4]. Later stages of the disease show a reduced number of follicular units and interstitial fibrosis [4]. A direct immunofluorescence test shows immunoglobulin G and complement C3 depositions along the basement membrane zone of both cutaneous and follicular epithelium. Antinuclear antibody titers are positive in 15–45% of cases. Treatment of discoid lupus erythematosus includes photoprotection, topical and oral corticosteroids, antimalarias, methotrexate, mycophenolate mofetil, azathioprine, dapsone, thalidomide, oral retinoids or in an extensive course of the disease- rituximab [6].

Differential diagnoses for the presented patient included lichen planopilaris, pseudopelade of Brocq and Brunsting-Perry cicatricial pemphigoid.

Lichen planopilaris is the most common cause of cicatricial alopecia. The disease most commonly affects women between 40 and 60 years of age. Typically, the vertex and parietal areas are involved. Lichen planopilaris presents as a hair loss area with the presence of perifollicular erythema and follicular hyperkeratosis at the periphery [4]. The lesions are commonly associated with itching, burning sensation and scalp tenderness.

Pseudopelade of Brocq is a chronic form of primary lymphocytic cicatricial alopecia. There are some controversies whether the disease is a final stage of other forms of scarring alopecia or a distinct clinicopathological entity. It is characterized by multiple, small, noninflammatory, white alopecic patches, resembling 'footprints on the snow', primarily located on the central scalp [4, 7].

Brunsting-Perry cicatricial pemphigoid is a chronic inflammatory, autoimmune condition. It is characterized by subepithelial blisters and erosions with following scarring strictly limited to the head and neck, sparing the mucous membranes [8].

Based on the clinical, trichoscopic and histopathological findings, the presented patient was diagnosed with discoid lupus erythematosus. The patient was treated with topical mometasone furoate and oral hydroxychloroquine 250 mg daily.

Key Points
- Discoid lupus erythematosus is a form of primary lymphocytic scarring alopecia
- The disease presents as discoid, well-circumscribed, erythematosus plaques with adherent follicular hyperkeratosis

References

1. Fabbri P, Amato L, Chiarini C, Moretti S, Massi D. Scarring alopecia in discoid lupus erythematosus: a clinical, histopathologic and immunopathologic study. Lupus. 2014;13(6):455–62.
2. Bolduc D, Sperling LC, Shapiro J. Primary cicatricial alopecia. J Am Acad Dermatol. 2016;75(6):1081–99.
3. Hordinsky M. Cicatricial alopecia: discoid lupus erythematosus. Dermatol Ther. 2008;21(4):245–8.
4. Concha JSS, Werth VP. Alopecias in lupus erythematosus. Lupus Sci Med. 2018;5:e000291.
5. Żychowska M, Żychowska M. Dermoscopy of discoid lupus erythematosus – a systematic review of the literature. Int J Dermatol. 2021;60(7):818–28. https://doi.org/10.1111/ijd.15365.
6. Ioannides D, Tosti A. Alopecias – practical evaluation and management. Curr Probl Dermatol. Basel, Karger. 2015;47:159–64.
7. Alzolibani AA, Kang H, Otberg N, Shapiro J. Pseudopelade of Brocq. Dermatol Ther. 2008;21(4):257–63. https://doi.org/10.1111/j.1529-8019.2008.00207.x.
8. Das S, Blanco G, Ahmed A, Tran KT, Matthews LA, Pandya AG. Cicatricial pemphigoid of the scalp mimicking discoid lupus erythematosus. J Am Acad Dermatol. 2011;65(4):886–7.

Chapter 10
A 62-Year-Old Woman with Mild Hair Loss and Scalp Itching

Anna Waśkiel-Burnat, Joanna Czuwara, Małgorzata Olszewska, and Lidia Rudnicka

A 62-year-old woman presented with a history of scalp itching and an increased hair loss since six months. There was no seasonal variation. No personal or family history of dermatologic diseases was reported.

A physical examination showed a mild scalp erythema and diffuse hair thinning (Fig. 10.1). There was no other skin, mucous membranes or nails lesions detected. On trichoscopic examination, a diffuse erythema and perifollicular scaling were observed (Fig. 10.2).

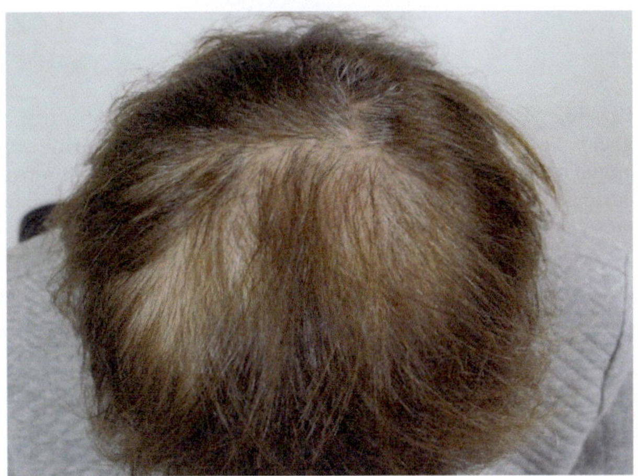

Fig. 10.1 A 62-year-old woman with a mild scalp erythema and diffuse hair thinning

A. Waśkiel-Burnat (✉) · J. Czuwara · M. Olszewska · L. Rudnicka
Department of Dermatology, Medical University of Warsaw, Warsaw, Poland
e-mail: anna.waskiel@wum.edu.pl; joanna.czuwara@wum.edu.pl; malgorzata.olszewska@wum.edu.pl; lidia.rudnicka@wum.edu.pl

A. Waśkiel-Burnat et al. (eds.), *Clinical Cases in Hair Disorders*, Clinical Cases in Dermatology, https://doi.org/10.1007/978-3-030-93423-1_10

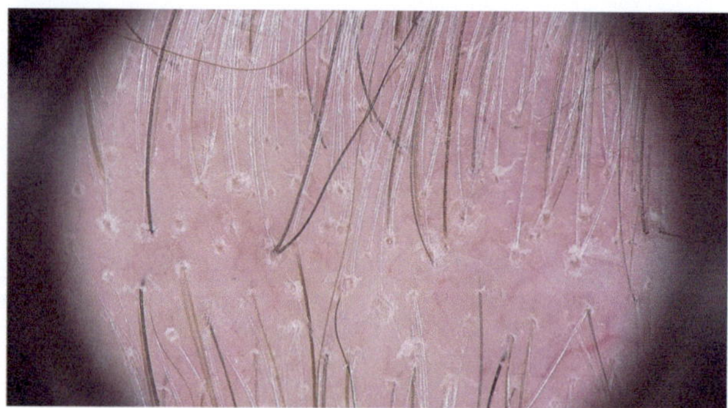

Fig. 10.2 Trichoscopy of the occipital area with the presence of dissuse erythema and perifollicular scaling (×20)

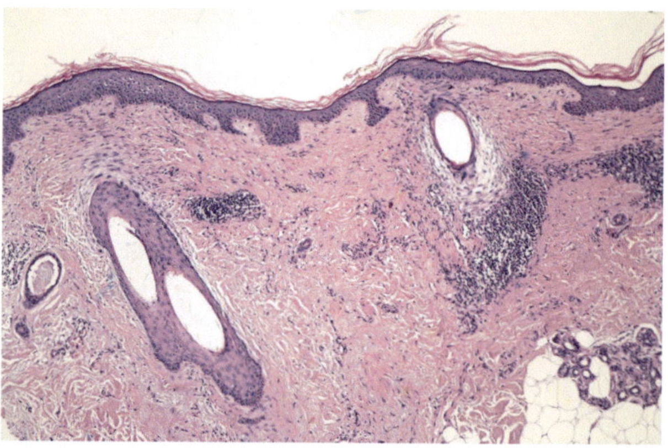

Fig. 10.3 Histopathology with the reduction of the number of terminal hair and loss of sebaceous glands and vellus follicles. Moreover hair follicles miniaturization with irregular and atrophic epithelia contracted by surrounding mucinous lamellar fibroplasia are observed. Fusion of the adjacent thinning follicular infundibula is visible. A lymphocytic inflammatory infiltrate is presented

Histopathology showed reduction of the number of terminal hair, loss of sebaceous glands and vellus follicles as well as lymphocytic inflammatory infiltrate (Fig. 10.3).

Based on the case description and the photographs, what is your diagnosis?

Differential Diagnoses

1. Seborrheic dermatitis.
2. Psoriasis.
3. Female androgenetic alopecia.
4. Lichen planopilaris diffuse pattern.

Diagnosis

Lichen planopilaris diffuse pattern.

Discussion

Lichen planopilaris, a follicular variant of lichen planus, is the most common cause of primary cicatricial alopecia [1]. Recently, a new variant of the disease was described and named as lichen planopilaris diffuse pattern [2]. Clinically, it is characterized by the presence of mild hair thinning with coexisted erythema and moderate to severe itching or burning sensation [2]. On trichoscopy, typical features of lichen planopilaris are presented and include perifollicular erythema, perifollicular scaling, red and milky-red areas with the absence of hair follicle openings [2]. In majority of cases, a trichoscopy-guided biopsy is mandatory to confirm the diagnosis [2]. A histological examination is characterized by the presence of a subepidermal interface dermatitis with lymphocytic infiltration of the infundibulum and isthmus of the hair follicle [2, 3]. Topical corticosteroids are recommended as the first-line therapy for lichen planopilaris diffuse pattern [2]. Other treatment options include systemic steroids, antimalarials, finasteride, retinoids, cyclosporine, mycophenolate mofetil and tetracycline/doxycycline [4].

Differential diagnoses for lichen planopilaris diffuse pattern are seborrheic dermatitis, psoriasis, and androgenetic alopecia.

Seborrheic dermatitis is a chronic inflammatory dermatologic condition. It presents as well-delimited erythematous plaques with greasy-looking, yellowish scales [5]. The scalp is most commonly affected, however the disease can appear also on the other body areas such as the face, chest, back, axilla, and groin [5, 6]. Itching sensation is usually presented [6]. Seborrheic dermatitis is characterized by a seasonal pattern, presenting more frequently during winter, and improving usually during summer [5].

Psoriasis is a chronic inflammatory dermatologic condition that affects mainly the extensor surface of elbows and knees, the scalp, and lower back. Scalp psoriasis is characterized by red, thickened plaques with silver-white scale, either contained within the hairline, or extending onto the forehead, ears, and posterior neck. In many cases, severe itch occurs [7].

Androgenetic alopecia, also known as pattern hair loss, is the most common form of non-scarring hair loss, characterized by a progressive miniaturization of terminal scalp hair with a pattern distribution [1]. In men, the vertex and frontotemporal areas are most prominently affected. In women, diffuse central thinning with the frontal hair line spared, prominent frontal scalp thinning with a Christmas tree-like pattern or recession of the hairline along the bilateral temporal regions is observed [8]. In androgenetic alopecia, an erythema, scaling and itching are no typical presented.

In the presented patient, based on the clinical manifestation, trichoscopic and histopathological findings the diagnosis of lichen planopilaris diffuse pattern was established. Treatment with topical clobetasol propionate and hydroxychloroquine (200 mg twice a day) was initiated. Reduction of the scalp erythema and perifollicular scaling was achieved.

Key Points

- In patients with diffuse hair thinning and a history of scalp erythema and itching lichen planopilaris diffuse pattern should be considered
- Trichoscopic features of lichen planopilaris diffuse pattern are perifollicular erythema, perifollicular scaling, red and milky-red areas with loss of hair follicle openings
- A trichoscopy-guided biopsy is useful to confirm the initial diagnosis

References

1. Vano-Galvan S, Saceda-Corralo D, Blume-Peytavi U, Cucchia J, Dlova NC, Gavazzoni Dias MFR, et al. Frequency of the types of alopecia at twenty-two specialist hair clinics: a multicenter study. Skin Appendage Disord. 2019;5(5):309–15.
2. Starace M, Orlando G, Alessandrini A, Baraldi C, Bruni F, Piraccini BM. Diffuse variants of scalp lichen planopilaris: clinical, trichoscopic, and histopathologic features of 40 patients. J Am Acad Dermatol. 2020;83(6):1659–67.
3. Kanti V, Rowert-Huber J, Vogt A, Blume-Peytavi U. Cicatricial alopecia. J Dtsch Dermatol Ges. 2018;16(4):435–61.
4. Errichetti E, Figini M, Croatto M, Stinco G. Therapeutic management of classic lichen planopilaris: a systematic review. Clin Cosmet Investig Dermatol. 2018;11:91–102.
5. Clark GW, Pope SM, Jaboori KA. Diagnosis and treatment of seborrheic dermatitis. Am Fam Physician. 2015;91(3):185–90.
6. Borda LJ, Wikramanayake TC. Seborrheic dermatitis and dandruff: a comprehensive review. J Clin Investig Dermatol. 2015;3(2) https://doi.org/10.13188/2373-1044.1000019.
7. Blakely K, Gooderham M. Management of scalp psoriasis: current perspectives. Psoriasis (Auckl). 2016;6:33–40.
8. Starace M, Orlando G, Alessandrini A, Piraccini BM. Female androgenetic alopecia: an update on diagnosis and management. Am J Clin Dermatol. 2020;21(1):69–84.

Chapter 11
A 64-Year-Old Woman with Burning Sensation of the Scalp with Coexisted Hair Loss

Anna Waśkiel-Burnat, Anna Stochmal, Małgorzata Olszewska, and Lidia Rudnicka

A 64-year-old woman presented with a seven-month history of burning sensation of the scalp with coexisted hair loss. No history of dermatologic diseases was reported.

A physical examination revealed area of scarring hair loss (4 cm × 4 cm) with perifollicular scaling and erythema at the periphery on the vertex area of the scalp (Fig. 11.1). No other skin, mucous membranes or nails lesions as well as hair loss in other hair-bearing areas were detected. On trichoscopic examination, perifollicular scaling, pili torti and white dots were observed. Moreover, milky-red and white areas with lack of follicular openings were detected (Fig. 11.2).

Based on the case description and the photographs, what is your diagnosis?

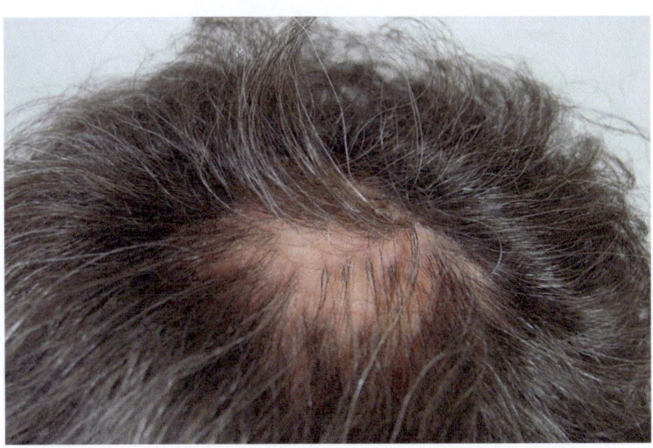

Fig. 11.1 A 64-year-old woman with scarring alopecia on the vertex area. Perifollicular scaling and erythema at the periphery are observed

A. Waśkiel-Burnat (✉) · A. Stochmal · M. Olszewska · L. Rudnicka
Department of Dermatology, Medical University of Warsaw, Warsaw, Poland
e-mail: anna.waskiel@wum.edu.pl; anna.stochmal@wum.edu.pl; malgorzata.olszewska@wum.edu.pl; lidia.rudnicka@wum.edu.pl

43

A. Waśkiel-Burnat et al. (eds.), *Clinical Cases in Hair Disorders*, Clinical Cases in Dermatology, https://doi.org/10.1007/978-3-030-93423-1_11

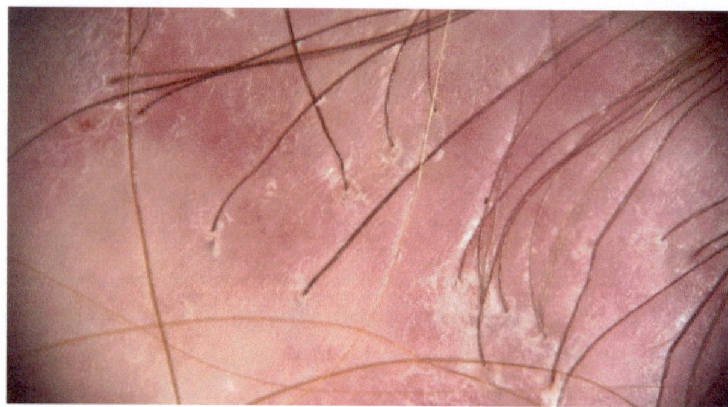

Fig. 11.2 Trichoscopy with the presence of perifollicular scaling, pili torti and milky-red areas with loss of follicular openings (×70)

Differential Diagnoses

1. Classic lichen planopilaris.
2. Discoid lupus erythematosus.
3. Pseudopelade of Brocq.
4. Central centrifugal cicatricial alopecia.

Diagnosis

Classic lichen planopilaris.

Discussion

Lichen planopilaris, a variant of lichen planus, is the primary lymphocyte-mediated form of scarring alopecia. The pathogenesis of the disease is not fully elucidated. However, an autoimmune etiology is suggested [1, 2]. Clinically, various subtypes of the disease are described: classic lichen planopilaris, frontal fibrosing alopecia and Graham-Little-Piccardi-Lassueur syndrome. Classic lichen planopilaris most commonly affects women between 40 and 60 years of age. It presents as areas of cicatricial hair loss with perifollicular erythema and follicular hyperkeratosis at the periphery that predominantly affect the vertex and parietal areas [3]. The lesions are commonly associated with itching, burning sensation and scalp tenderness. The diagnosis of classic lichen planopilaris is established based on the clinical picture and histopathological examination. Trichoscopy may be useful to avoid the scalp biopsy. Trichoscopic features of lichen planopilaris are perifollicular scaling, perifollicular erythema, white and blue-grey dots, milky-red areas and white areas lacking of follicular openings [3]. In histopathological examination, a dense lymphocytic infiltrate and fibrosis around the infundibulum and isthmus of the hair follicle with lichenoid interface dermatitis involving the upper follicle and loss of sebaceous glands are observed [2]. Topical corticosteroids and intralesional corticosteroid injections are usually the first-line therapy for classic lichen planopilaris. Other treatment options include systemic steroids, antimalarials, retinoids, cyclosporine, mycophenolate mofetil and tetracycline/doxycycline [4].

Differential diagnoses for included discoid lupus erythematosus, pseudopelade of Brocq and central centrifugal cicatricial alopecia.

Discoid lupus erythematosus, a variant of chronic cutaneous lupus erythematosus, is a form of lymphocytic primary cicatricial alopecia. Typically, it occurs in women between 20 and 40 years of age. The disease is characterized by circumscribed erythematous indurated plaques with coexisted scaling. When the adherent scale is removed, follicular plugging may be observed (carpet tack sign). Telangiectasias, atrophy, depigmentation, and hyperpigmentation may be detected [2]. Unlike lichen planopilaris, the inflammatory lesions of discoid lupus erythematosus are usually presented within the alopecic patches rather than at the periphery [1].

Pseudopelade of Brocq is a form of lymphocytic primary scarring alopecia characterized by the presence of multiple small flash-toned alopecic areas with irregular borders without hyperkeratosis and inflammatory signs (sometimes reminiscent of "footprints in the snow"). It most commonly affects women between the ages of 30 and 50. The lesions are usually localized on the vertex and the parietal areas [1, 2].

Central centrifugal cicatricial alopecia is a form of primary lymphocytic cicatricial alopecia that mainly affects women of African descent. The disease is characterized by a single area of cicatricial alopecia on the vertex area with slow, often symmetric peripheral progression. Perifollicular hyperpigmentation, erythema, polytrichia and islands of unaffected skin within the affected area are observed. Pruritus and burning sensation are usually reported [1, 2].

In the present patient, based on the clinical manifestation and trichoscopic features, the diagnosis of classic lichen planopilaris was established. Treatment with acitretin (20 mg daily) with intralesional triamcinolone acetonide (10 mg/ml) every four to six weeks was started.

Key Points
- Lichen planopilaris is the most common cause of primary cicatricial alopecia
- Characteristic features of lichen planopilaris are perifollicular erythema and perifollicular scaling

References

1. Kanti V, Rowert-Huber J, Vogt A, Blume-Peytavi U. Cicatricial alopecia. J Dtsch Dermatol Ges. 2018;16(4):435–61.

2. Fanti PA, Baraldi C, Misciali C, Piraccini BM. Cicatricial alopecia. G Ital Dermatol Venereol. 2018;153(2):230–42.
3. Waśkiel A, Rakowska A, Sikora M, Olszewska M, Rudnicka L. Trichoscopy in lichen planopilaris: an update. Dermatology Review/Przegląd Dermatologiczny. 2018;105(1):63–75.
4. Errichetti E, Figini M, Croatto M, Stinco G. Therapeutic management of classic lichen planopilaris: a systematic review. Clin Cosmet Investig Dermatol. 2018;11:91–102.

Chapter 12
A 66-Year-Old Woman with Localized Hair Loss

Anna Waśkiel-Burnat, Joanna Czuwara, Małgorzata Olszewska, and Lidia Rudnicka

A 66-year-old woman presented with a two-month history of localized hair loss with coexisted itch. The patient had hypertension, type 2 diabetes mellitus and hyperlipidemia. No history of dermatologic or hematological diseases was reported.

A physical examination revealed an erythematous plaque (10 cm × 5 cm) with coexisted non-scarring hair loss on the vertex and occipital areas (Fig. 12.1). On trichoscopic examination, yellow dots and single exclamation mark hairs, Pohl-Pinkus constrictions, black dots and upgrowing hairs were presented. Additionally,

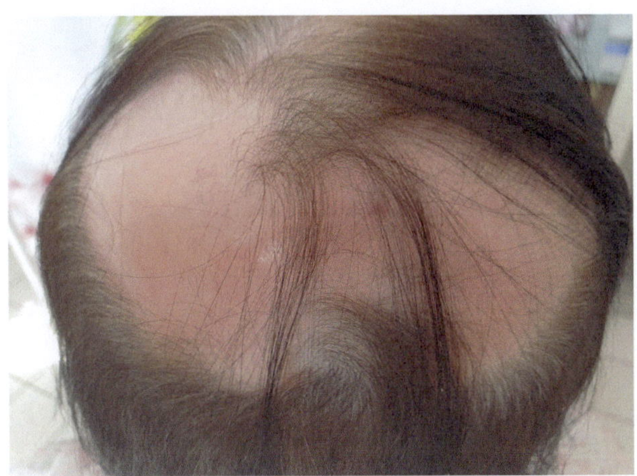

Fig. 12.1 A 66-year-old woman with an erythematous plaque and coexisted non-scarring hair loss on the vertex and occipital areas

A. Waśkiel-Burnat (✉) · J. Czuwara · M. Olszewska · L. Rudnicka
Department of Dermatology, Medical University of Warsaw, Warsaw, Poland
e-mail: anna.waskiel@wum.edu.pl; joanna.czuwara@wum.edu.pl;
malgorzata.olszewska@wum.edu.pl; lidia.rudnicka@wum.edu.pl

A. Waśkiel-Burnat et al. (eds.), *Clinical Cases in Hair Disorders*, Clinical Cases in Dermatology, https://doi.org/10.1007/978-3-030-93423-1_12

"""

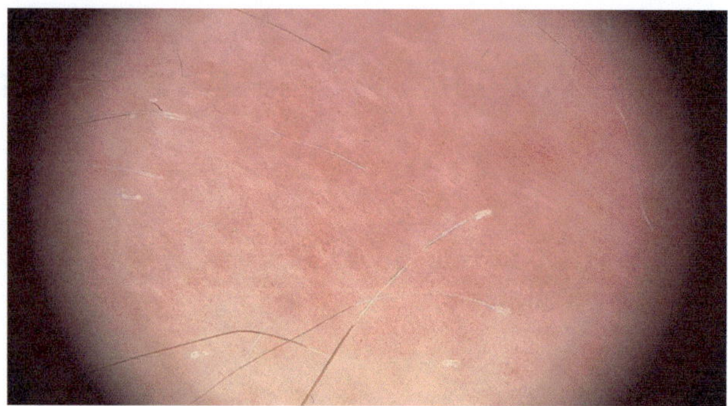

Fig. 12.2 Trichoscopy with the presence of perifollicular scaling, white lines, dotted and linear vessels (×20)

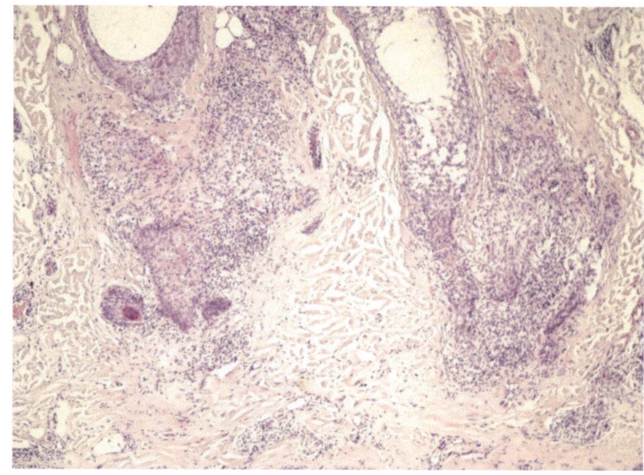

Fig. 12.3 Histopathology with the presence of peribulbar lymphocytic infiltrate and mucin depositions within the hair follicle

perifollicular scaling, dotted vessels, linear vessels and white lines were observed (Fig. 12.2).

A histopathological examination shows a peribulbar lymphocytic infiltrate as well as mucin depositions within the hair follicles and sebaceous glands (Fig. 12.3). Immunohistochemistry showed normal CD4 to CD8 ratio and CD5 and CD7 expression.

Based on the case description and the photographs, what is your diagnosis?

Differential Diagnoses

1. Mycosis fungoides.
2. Alopecia areata.
3. Follicular mucinosis.
4. Tinea capitis.

Diagnosis

Follicular mucinosis coexisted with alopecia areata.

Discussion

Follicular mucinosis, also known as alopecia mucinosa, is a form of cutaneous mucinosis characterized by accumulation of dermal type mucin in the pilosebaceous follicle and sebaceous glands [1]. Pathogenesis of the disease is not fully understood. There are two main clinicopathological forms of follicular mucinosis: a primary and a secondary form associated with benign or malignant condition [1]. The secondary form of follicular mucinosis is most commonly associated with mycosis fungoides. Other lymphoproliferative disorders are also common and include Sezary syndrome, Hodgkin's lymphoma, chronic lymphocytic leukemia, cutaneous B-cell lymphoma, acute myelogenous leukemia, adult T-cell leukemia–lymphoma, and chronic myelomonocytic leukemia. They may precede, arise with, or follow the diagnosis. Secondary follicular mucinosis has been also described in multiple inflammatory or infectious conditions such as demodicosis, eosinophilic folliculitis, insect or tick bite. Other cutaneous conditions which may be associated with the disease are seborrheic keratosis, simple prurigo, acne vulgaris, polymorphous light eruption, drug-related vasculitis, atopic dermatitis and systemic lupus erythematosus [1]. Coexistence of follicular mucinosis with alopecia areata has been rarely described [2]. Secondary follicular mucinosis mainly affects elderly. Clinically, it is characterized by the presence of well-delimited, erythematous or brownish-erythematous papules or plaques. Follicular keratosis or areas of alopecia may be presented. Hair loss in the course of follicular mucinosis is typically non-scarring and reversible; in very rare cases, scarring may occur [3]. The disease can be observed in any body area, however the scalp, neck and upper extremities are most commonly affected [1]. The diagnosis of follicular mucinosis is based on the clinicopathologic correlation. In histopathological examination mucin deposits on the outer root sheath of the hair follicle, in addition to inflammatory infiltrates composed of lymphocytes, macrophages and eosinophils with folliculotropic lymphocytes are presented [4]. Additionally, immunohistochemical and molecular studies are necessary to diagnose underlying condition. Similar modalities have also been used in the treatment of both, primary and secondary folliculitis mucinosis. Therapeutic options include mild-to-moderate potency topical corticosteroids, topical and oral antibiotics, retinoids, dapsone, imiquimod, pimecrolimus, and psoralen plus ultraviolet A (PUVA). Moreover, in a secondary form therapy should target the underlying cause.

Differential diagnoses for the presented patient included mycosis fungoides, tinea capitis and alopecia areata.

Mycosis fungoides is the most common type of primary cutaneous T-cell lymphoma. It occurs more frequently in older adults and is more commonly observed in men compared to women. There are three main stages of cutaneous involvement of mucosis fungoides: patchy-, plaque-, and tumor-stage. Lesions affects mainly photo-protected areas, in particular the buttocks, groin, breasts, upper thighs, and axilla and, less commonly, the distal extremities, head, and neck [4].

Another differential diagnosis is tinea capitis, a fungal infection of the scalp that affects mainly children. The disease is characterized by the presence of hair loss areas with coexistent scaling, inflammation or pustules [5]. Itch is usually reported [6].

Alopecia areata, a form of non-scarring autoimmune hair loss, is characterized by the presence of hair loss areas within the skin which remains normal. Although the scalp is the most commonly affected, hair loss can also be observed in other hair-bearing areas (such as eyebrows, eyelashes, pubic and axillary areas) [7]. Trichoscopic features of alopecia areata are black dots, broken hairs, exclamation mark hairs, tapered hairs, vellus hairs, yellow dots, upright regrowing hairs, pigtail (circle) hairs, and Pohl-Pinkus constrictions.

In the presented patient, based on the clinical, trichoscopic and histopathological examinations the diagnosis of secondary follicular mucinosis with coexisted alopecia areata was established. Clobetasol propionate 0.05% cream once a day was recommended. Reduction of erythema and partial hair regrowth was observed.

Key Points
- Secondary follicular mucinosis is associated with various malignant or benign conditions (e.g. alopecia areata)
- The disease is characterized by the presence of well-delimited, erythematous or brownish-erythematous papules or plaques
- Follicular keratosis and non-scarring hair loss may be observed

References

1. Khalil J, Kurban M, Abbas O. Follicular mucinosis: a review. Int J Dermatol. 2021;60:159–65.
2. Fanti PA, Tosti A, Morelli R, Cameli N, Sabattini E, Pileri S. Follicular mucinosis in alopecia areata. Am J Dermatopathol. 1992;14(6):542–5.
3. Kanti V, Rowert-Huber J, Vogt A, Blume-Peytavi U. Cicatricial alopecia. J Dtsch Dermatol Ges. 2018;16(4):435–61.
4. Pincus LB. Mycosis Fungoides. Surg Pathol Clin. 2014;7(2):143–67.
5. Adesiji YO, Omolade FB, Aderibigbe IA, Ogungbe O, Adefioye OA, Adedokun SA, et al. Prevalence of tinea capitis among children in Osogbo, Nigeria, and the associated risk factors. Diseases. 2019;7(1)
6. Rudnicka L, Olszewska M, Rakowska A. Atlas of Trichocopy: dermoscopy in hair and scalp disease. London: Springer; 2012.
7. Waskiel A, Rakowska A, Sikora M, Olszewska M, Rudnicka L. Trichoscopy of alopecia areata: an update. J Dermatol. 2018;45(6):692–700.

Chapter 13
A 70-Year-Old Woman with Areas of Scarring Hair Loss

Agata Szykut-Badaczewska and Mariusz Sikora

A 70-year-old woman presented with patchy alopecia on the scalp. The first area of hair loss occurred on the vertex four years ago. Within the last year, a new area of hair loss on the occipital region has developed. The patient had hypertension and hypothyroidism. No personal or family history of dermatological disorders was reported.

A physical examination revealed two foci of scarring alopecia on the vertex (Fig. 13.1) and the occipital scalp (Fig. 13.2). On trichoscopy of the vertex lesion,

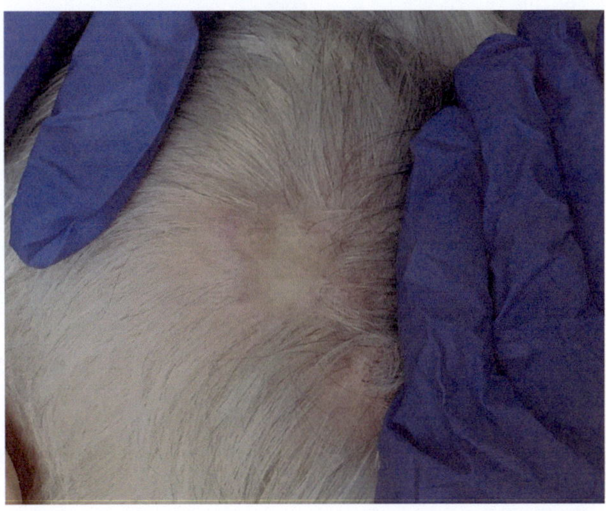

Fig. 13.1 A 70-year-old woman with area of scarring hair loss on the vertex area since 4 years

A. Szykut-Badaczewska (✉) · M. Sikora
Department of Dermatology, Medical University of Warsaw, Warsaw, Poland
e-mail: agata.szykut-badaczewska@wum.edu.pl; mariusz.sikora@spartanska.pl

A. Waśkiel-Burnat et al. (eds.), *Clinical Cases in Hair Disorders*, Clinical Cases in Dermatology, https://doi.org/10.1007/978-3-030-93423-1_13

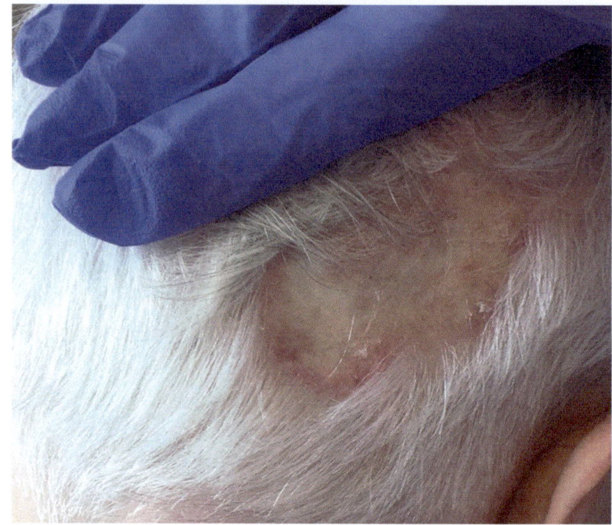

Fig. 13.2 Newly developed area of scarring hair loss on the occipital area

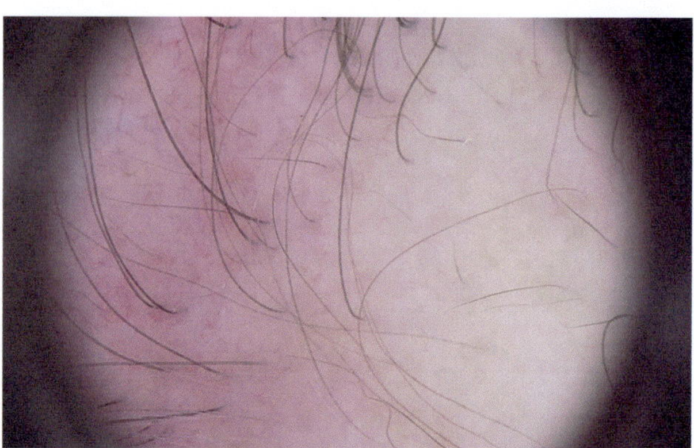

Fig. 13.3 Trichoscopy of the lesion on the vertex area with the presence of porcelain-white, avascular area surrounded by thin arborizing vessels was observed (x20)

diffuse, porcelain-white, avascular area surrounded by thin arborizing vessels was observed (Fig. 13.3). Trichoscopy of the occipital lesion showed large yellow dots, red dots, diffuse brown discoloration and thick arborizing vessels (Fig. 13.4). Punch biopsies from two lesions were performed.

A histopathological examination of the vertex lesion showed thickening of collagen fibers in the reticular layer of the dermis. In histopathological examination of the occipital lesion, a periadnexal, lymphocytic inflammatory infiltrate reaching the adipose tissue with features of fibrosis were observed. A direct immunofluorescence test revealed linear deposits of IgM and IgG immunoglobulins at the basement membrane zone. Antinuclear antibodies titers were positive.

Based on the case description and the photographs, what is your diagnosis?

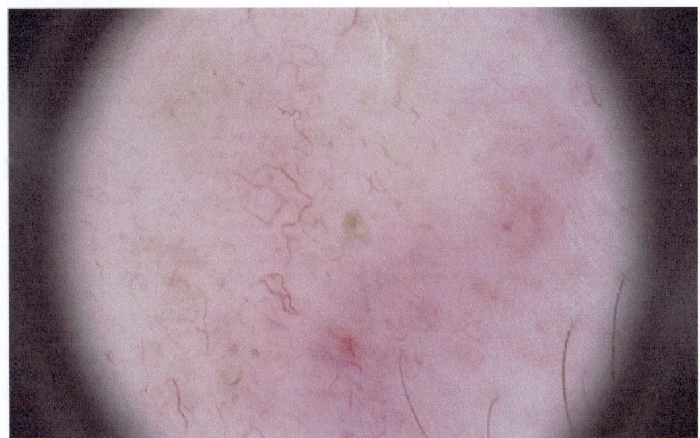

Fig. 13.4 Trichoscopy of the lesion on the occipital area showed large yellow dots, red dots, diffuse brown discoloration and thick arborizing vessels (x20)

Differential Diagnoses

1. Lichen planopilaris.
2. Discoid lupus erythematosus.
3. Morphea (localized scleroderma).
4. Pseudopelade of Brocq.

Diagnosis

Morphea with discoid lupus erythematosus.

Discussion

Morphea, also known as localized scleroderma, is a rare inflammatory disease of the skin and subcutaneous tissue. The pathogenesis of the disease is unknown, but the role of genetic predisposition, autoimmune dysregulation, and environmental factors is suggested. The incidence rate of morphea varies from 3.4 to 27 per 100,000. The condition is more common in women and usually occurs in the fourth decade of life [1]. Children are also commonly affected, mainly between seven and 11 years of age. The disease involves a wide variety of clinical phenotypes such as circumscribed, linear, generalized, pansclerotic and mixed [1]. Circumscribed morphea is the most common variant that is characterized by the isolated oval or round lesions mainly localized on the trunk. The scalp involvement is rarely observed. Early lesions of morphea present as an erythema and induration with some itching and tenderness. As the lesions progress, they develop sclerotic centres surrounded by a violaceous border. The lesions result in hyperpigmentation or hypopigmentation with atrophy of the skin and subcutaneous tissue. Coexistence of morphea with discoid lupus erythematosus has been rarely described in the literature. Morphea is usually diagnosed clinically. Dermoscopic and histopathological examinations are helpful to confirm the diagnosis. Dermoscopic findings of morphea are whitish areas crossed by linear branching vessels [2]. Histopathology of localised scleroderma depends on the stage of the disease. In early, active lesions, a perivascular infiltrate, predominantly composed of lymphocytes and plasma cells with some eosinophils and macrophages are observed. Older sclerotic lesions demonstrate collagen bundles extending into the reticular dermis, enclosing the eccrine glands and blood vessels [1]. Topical corticosteroids are usually the first-line treatment for superficial morphea. Topical tacrolimus 0.1% is an alternative choice. For patients with more widespread lesions and deep morphea, the first-line treatment is phototherapy. Rapidly progressive lesions require systemic therapy with corticosteroids or methotrexate. Mycophenolate mofetil may also be useful [1].

Differential diagnoses for the presented patient included discoid lupus erythematosus, lichen planopilaris and pseudopelade of Brocq.

Lichen planopilaris is the most common cause of cicatricial alopecia. The disease most commonly affects women, between 40 and 60 years of age. Typically, the vertex and parietal areas are involved. Lichen planopilaris presents as an area of hair loss with the presence of perifollicular erythema and follicular hyperkeratosis at the periphery [3, 4].

Discoid lupus erythematosus, a variant of chronic cutaneous lupus erythematosus, is a form of lymphocytic primary cicatricial alopecia. Typically, it occurs in women between 20 and 40 years of age. Discoid lupus erythematosus presents as circumscribed indurated plaques with coexisting scaling. When the adherent scale is removed, follicular plugging may be observed (carpet tack sign). Telangiectasias, atrophy, depigmentation, and hyperpigmentation may be detected [4].

Pseudopelade of Brocq is a form of lymphocytic primary scarring alopecia characterized by the presence of multiple small flash-toned alopecic areas with irregular borders without hyperkeratosis and inflammatory signs (sometimes reminiscent of "footprints on the snow"). It most commonly affects women between the age of 30 and 50 years. The lesions are usually localized on the vertex and parietal areas [3, 4].

Based on the clinical, trichoscopic and histopathological features, the diagnosis of morphea with discoid lupus erythematosus was established [5]. The patient was started on oral methotrexate 15 mg once a week and mometasone furoate ointment once daily. No hair loss progression was observed six months after the treatment initiation.

Key Points

- Circumscribed morphea is the most common variant that rarely affects the scalp area
- Initially morphea presents as an erythematous plaque; with progression sclerotic centre surrounded by a violaceous border is observed

- The lesion results in hyper- or hypopigmentation with atrophy of the skin and subcutaneous tissue
- Morphea may coexist with discoid lupus erythematosus

References

1. Penmetsa GK, Sapra A. Morphea. 2020 Aug 10. In: StatPearls. Treasure Island (FL): StatPearls Publishing; 2020.
2. Errichetti E, Stinco G. Dermoscopy in general dermatology: a practical overview. Dermatol Ther (Heidelb). 2016;6(4):471–507.
3. Kanti V, Rowert-Huber J, Vogt A, Blume-Peytavi U. Cicatricial alopecia. J Dtsch Dermatol Ges. 2018;16(4):435–61.
4. Fanti PA, Baraldi C, Misciali C, Piraccini BM. Cicatricial alopecia. G Ital Dermatol Venereol. 2018;153(2):230–42.
5. Florez-Pollack S, Kunzler E, Jacobe HT. Morphea: current concepts. Clin Dermatol. 2018;36(4):475–86.

Chapter 14
A 70-Year-Old Woman with Non-tender Nodules with Coexisted Alopecia on the Scalp

Tatiana Silyuk

A 70-year-old woman presented with a ten-month history of asymptomatic nodules surrounded by erythematous, hairless areas on the scalp. The patient reported history of breast cancer diagnosed 14 years ago. The patient underwent surgery and chemotherapy with complete remission. She had regular follow up. Computed tomography scan of chest did not show any abnormalities.

A physical examination of the scalp revealed six firm, no-movable nodules surrounded by shinny an erythematous area with hair loss and telangiectasias (Figs. 14.1 and 14.2).

Trichoscopy revealed the absence of the hair follicles ostia and thick arborizing vessels (Fig. 14.3).

Based on the case description and the photographs, what is your diagnosis?

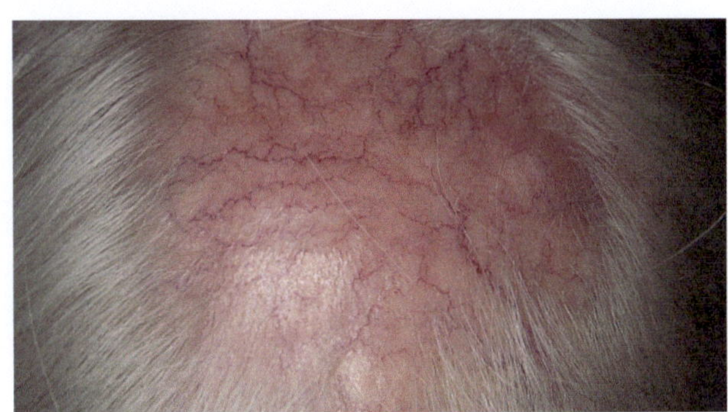

Fig. 14.1 A 70-year-old woman with nodules and a shiny erythematous area with hair loss and telangiectasias

T. Silyuk (✉)
Hair Care Center, Saint Petersburg, Russia

A. Waśkiel-Burnat et al. (eds.), *Clinical Cases in Hair Disorders*, Clinical Cases in Dermatology, https://doi.org/10.1007/978-3-030-93423-1_14

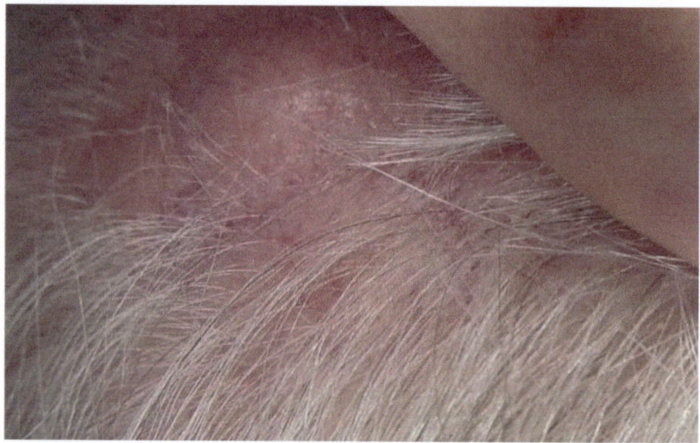

Fig. 14.2 A nodule surrounded by an erythematous area with coexisted hair loss

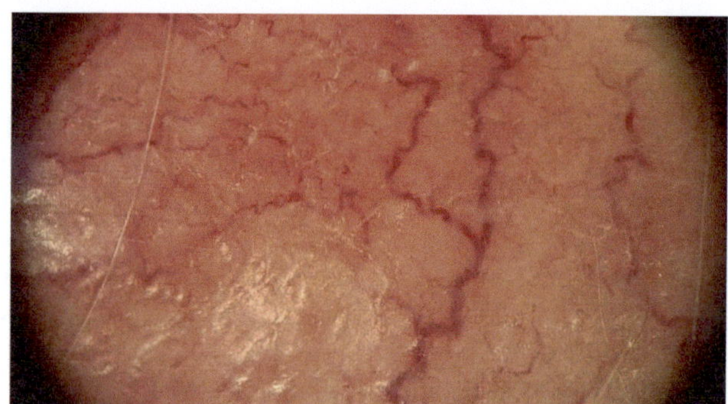

Fig. 14.3 Trichoscopy with the absence of the hair follicular ostia and thick arborizng vessels (×20)

Differential Diagnoses

1. Pilar cyst.
2. Scalp metastases (alopecia neoplastica).
3. Discoid lupus erythematosus.
4. Sarcoidosis.

Diagnosis

Scalp metastasis (alopecia neoplastica).

Discussion

Skin metastasis from primary visceral malignancy is uncommon clinical entity, with a reported incidence ranging from 0.22% to 12% of all malignancies. The most frequent areas of cutaneous metastases are the trunk, extremities, and perineum [1].

Breast cancer and melanoma are the most common cancers which spread to/within the skin. Other malignancies such as lung, colon and renal are also frequently implicated [1]. Skin metastasis may be the first sign of visceral tumors or it may occur many years after the diagnosis of malignancy. Clinically, skin metastases present as a single or multiple non-tender nodules which are characterized by rapid growth. Disfigurement, pain, bleeding, and drainage may occur [1].

The scalp is a common location for cutaneous metastases what may be explained by the higher blood supply of this area, compared to other body regions [2]. The scalp involvement is observed 4% to 7% of patients with skin metastases [2]. The primary sites of tumors with scalp metastases are usually the lungs, prostate, and breast [3].

Alopecia neoplastica is a pattern of scalp metastasis. The exact mechanism of the condition is still unknown. It has been suggested that hair loss is secondary to the dermal infiltration of tumor cells originating from a metastatic malignancy. It is unclear whether fibrosis or cytokine secretion from tumor cells leads to disappearance of the hair follicles [3]. Alopecia neoplastica presents as a hairless patch or a plaque with or without scaling. Subcutaneous nodule and teleangiectasia may be observed. Severe itching may be also reported.

The diagnosis of skin metastasis is established based on histopathological examination. Systemic chemotherapeutics targeting the primary tumor is the standard of care, but skin-directed therapies and immunotherapies may be also effective. The skin-directed therapeutic options include electrochemotherapy, photodynamic therapy, radiotherapy, intralesional therapy, and topical therapy [1].

Differential diagnoses for the presented patient were pilar cyst, discoid lupus erythematosus and sarcoidosis.

Pilar cyst is a form dermal cyst that arises from the epithelium located between the sebaceous gland and the arrector pili muscle. Pilar cysts are predominantly detected on the scalp and present as slow-growing, flesh-colored, smooth, mobile, firm, and well-circumscribed nodules. Most commonly, they are multiple lesions, but sometimes, single lesions might be presented. In case of long duration hair loss on the skin surface immediately above the cyst may be observed. The lesions are usually asymptomatic [4, 5].

Discoid lupus erythematosus is a form of lymphocytic primary cicatricial alopecia that occurs usually in women between 20 and 40 years of age. The disease is characterized by the circumscribed erythematous indurated plaques with coexisted scaling. When the adherent scale is removed, follicular plugging may be observed (carpet tack sign). Telangiectasias, atrophy, depigmentation, and hyperpigmentation may be detected. No nodular lesions are observed [6].

Sarcoidosis is a multisystem disorder of unknown etiology characterized by formation of non-caseating epithelioid granulomas. Sarcoidosis of the scalp is rarely reported. It presents as red-brown, violaceous or hypopigmented papules and plaques with nonscarring or rarely scarring hair loss. Skin lesions are usually associated with systemic involvement [7].

Based on the patient's history, clinical manifestation and trichoscopy, the diagnosis of scalp metastasis (alopecia neoplastica) was established. Skin punch biopsy with histopathological examination confirmed diagnosis of breast cancer metastasis.

Key Points

- In the case of nodular lesions on the scalp, skin metastates from primary visceral malignancy need to be excluded
- Alopecia neoplastica is a pattern of cutaneous metastasis to the scalp that is characterized by the presence of a hairless patch or a plaque with or without scaling

References

1. Strickley JD, Jenson AB, Jung JY. Cutaneous Metastasis. Hematol Oncol Clin North Am. 2019;33(1):173–97.
2. Kim J-H, Kim M-J, et al. Alopecia neoplastica due to gastric adenocarcinoma metastasis to the scalp, presenting as alopecia: a case report and literature review. Ann Dermatol. 2014;26(5):624–7.
3. Skafida E, Triantafyllopoulou I, Flessas I, et al. Secondary alopecia Neoplastica mimicking alopecia Areata following breast cancer. Case Rep Oncol. 2020;13:627–32.
4. Al Aboud DM, Yarrarapu SNS, Patel BC. Pilar cyst. StatPearls [Internet].
5. Leppard BJ, Sanderson KV. The natural history of trichilemmal cysts. Brit J Derm. 1976;94:379–90.
6. Kanti V, Rowert-Huber J, Vogt A, Blume-Peytavi U. Cicatricial alopecia. J Dtsch Dermatol Ges. 2018;16(4):435–61.
7. Katta R, Nelson B, et al. Sarcoidosis of the scalp: a case series and review of the literature. J Am Acad Dermatol. 2000;42:690–2.

Chapter 15
A Case of Alopecia

Pınar Ergen, Yasemin Yuyucu Karabulut, and Ümit Türsen

A 51-year-old male patient presented with erythematous, mildly scaly papules and plaques with coexisted scarring on the scalp, face and neck since one year (Fig. 15.1). Moreover, there was a hemorrhagic dried lesion on the lower lip since one month. A neurological examination and the other systemic examinations were normal. There were no laboratory abnormalities including complete blood count, biochemistry, urinanalysis, anti nuclear antibodies. In histopathological evaluation, orthokeratosis and follicular plugs in the epidermis were observed. Moreover, an accumulation of eosinophilic granular material, involving the dermoepidermal junction and superficial dermis, was noted. A perivascular and periadnexal mild lymphocyte infiltration in the superficial and deep dermis was observed (Fig. 15.2). A mucin accumulation between collagen fibers in the dermis, highlighted with periodic acid stain (PAS)- alcian blue was presented (Fig. 15.3). In direct immunofluorescence (DIF) examination, moderate granular accumulation of IgG, mild granular accumulation of IgA and mild linear accumulation of C3 were observed at the dermoepidermal junction (Fig. 15.4).

Based on the case description and the photograph, what is your diagnosis?

Differential Diagnoses

1. Discoid lupus erythematosus.
2. Subacute cutaneous lupus erythematosus.
3. Polymorphic light eruption.
4. Lichen planopilaris.

P. Ergen · Y. Y. Karabulut · Ü. Türsen (✉)
Department of Dermatology, Mersin University, School of Medicine, Mersin, Turkey
e-mail: pnryldrm8@mersin.edu.tr

© The Author(s), under exclusive license to Springer Nature Switzerland AG 2022

A. Waśkiel-Burnat et al. (eds.), *Clinical Cases in Hair Disorders*, Clinical Cases in Dermatology, https://doi.org/10.1007/978-3-030-93423-1_15

Fig. 15.1 Erythematous scaly lesions located on the scalp, forehead and face

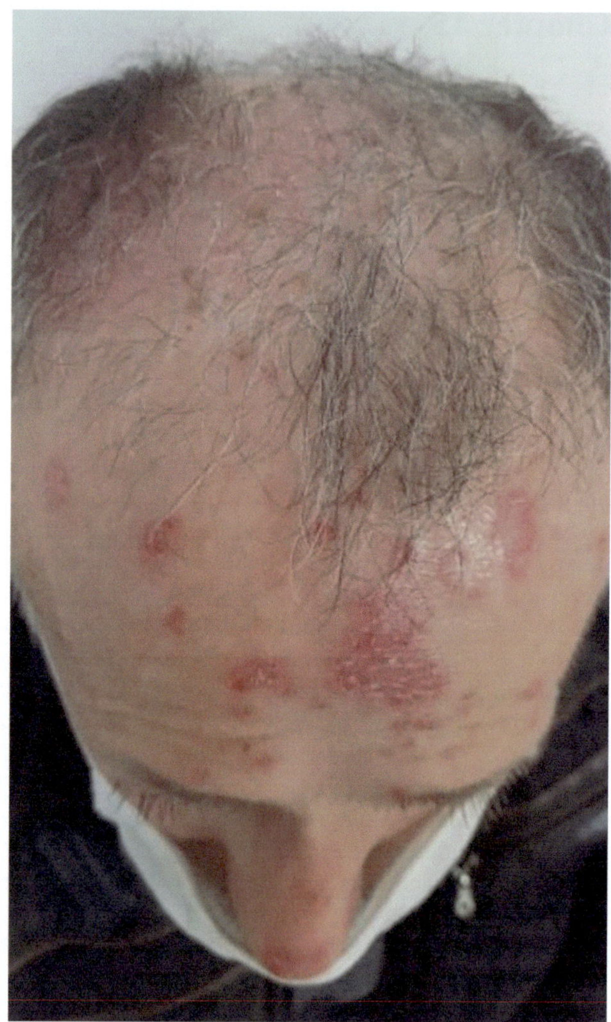

Diagnosis

Discoid lupus erythematosus.

Discussion

Lupus erythematosus (LE) is a systemic connective tissue disease characterized by the presence of pathogenic autoantibodies and immune complexes that cause loss of immune tolerance. Various forms of the cutaneous lesions in lupus

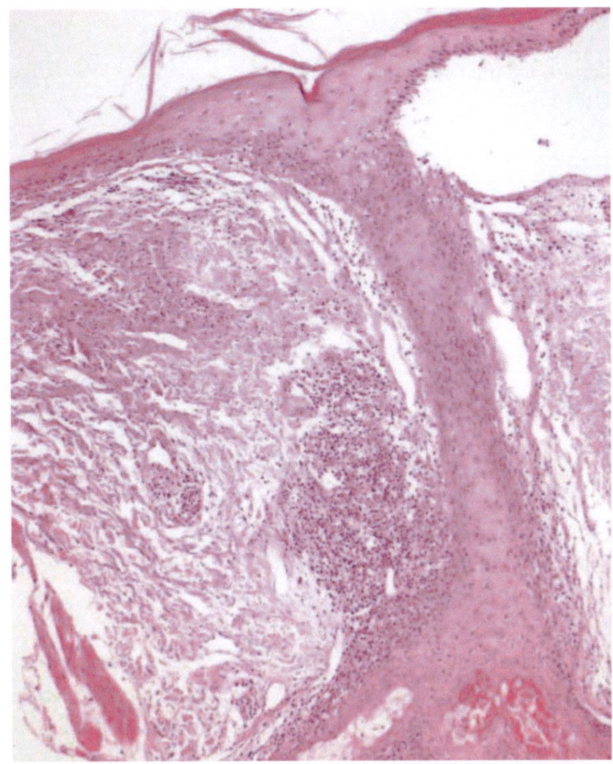

Fig. 15.2 Histology shows orthokeratosis, follicular plugging, eosinophilic granular material in the dermoepidermal junction, perivascular and periadnexal lymphoid infiltration in the superficial and deep dermis (H&E × 100)

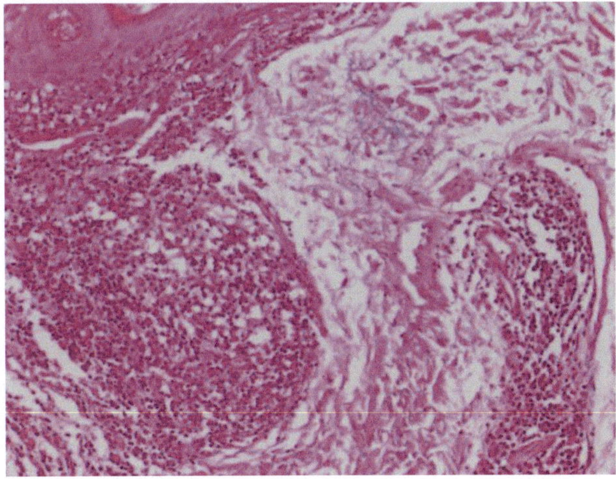

Fig. 15.3 A Perifollicular and perivascular lymphoid infiltration and dermal mucine accumulation (PAS - alcian blue ×200)

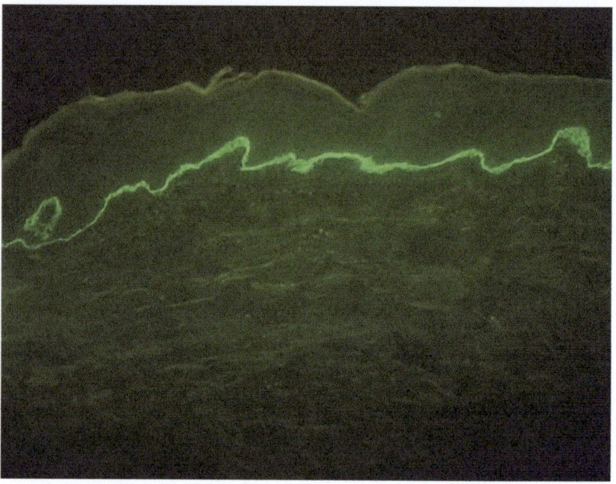

Fig. 15.4 A granular IgG accumulation at the dermoepidermal junction (IgG ×200)

erythematosus have been described. These are acute cutaneous lupus erythematosus (ACLE), subacute cutaneous lupus erythematosus (SCLE) and chronic cutaneous lupus erythematosus (CCLE) [1]. Discoid lupus erythematosus (DLE), the most common form of CCLE, can be localized or generalized. The number of lesions has prognostic significance. Only about 1% of patients with localized DLE develops systemic disease, but about 5% of patients with generalized form develops systemic manifestations. DLE lesions develop in up to 20% of patients with systemic lupus erythematosus [2].

DLE is more common in women in the fourth and fifth decades [1]. Localized lesions occur in areas that are frequently exposed to the sun, such as the face, head and neck. These light-sensitive lesions may be in the form of butterfly-like rash on the face. In the generalized form, areas not exposed to sunlight such as the trunk, upper extremities, palms and soles are also involved [3]. The lesions consist of sharp-edged, erythematous, scaly patches and plaques with telangiectasia [4].

Histopathologically, the epidermis and dermis are affected, while the subcutaneous tissue is usually preserved. Atrophy, hyperkeratosis, vacuolar degeneration in the basal layer, scattered apopitotic keratinocytes in the basal layer or epidermis as well as follicular plugs are observed. A perivascular and periadnexal lichenoid type or patchy infiltration consisting mostly of lymphocytes with less histiocyte can be seen in the dermis [4, 5]. While perivascular fibrin extravasation and edema are seen in an early period, thickening of the epidermal and follicular basement membranes and the wall of the capillaries is evident in long-standing lesions. Dermal fibroplasia and sometimes epidermal atrophy in long-term lesions may be also presented. Plasma cells may occur in the deep parts of the infiltration and are often presented in oral lesions. Eosinophils and neutrophils are usually absent. A dermal mucin accumulation is observed [6].

In histopathological examination, variable degrees of acanthosis in the epidermis are observed. A significant acanthosis is mainly seen in a hypertrophic variant of DLE that is often localized in the face and arm. The hypertrophic variants of DLE may be confused with keratoacanthoma and squamous cell carcinoma [3]. The histological features of tumid lupus erythematosus, which is another variant of DLE, coincide with polymorphic light eruption. Polymorphous light eruption, the most common photodermatosis, usually occurs as recurrent, erythematous papules, vesicles, and/or plaques on areas exposed to ultraviolet (UV) light in young people, especially women. Lesions heal without scars [7]. A dense perivascular lymphohistiocytic infiltrate, often associated with papillary dermal edema, is presented [8]. The presence of prominent papillary dermal edema is a typical sign of polymorphous light eruption; dermal mucin is not seen [8, 9].

Scalp involvement in DLE is commonly presented. Scaring alopecia develops due to follicular epithelial damage [10]. The most common cause of scaring alopecia is lichen planopilaris (LPP) [11]. In LPP, hyperkeratosis is presented on the periphery of the lesions, while in DLE it is observed in the central area [12]. In LPP, the infiltrate is mainly seen around the hair follicles [4]. A mucin deposits are not usually observed [12].

The histomorphological features of DLE overlap significantly with SCLE. The distinction between these two entities can be very difficult [4]. Contrary to DLE, hyperkeratosis, pilosebaceous atrophy, follicular plug formation, and basement membrane thickening in SCLE are less commonly observed; while atrophy, basal vacuolar change, dermal edema and mucin deposition are more prominent [4].

Lupus band test (LBT) is a diagnostic procedure used to detect immunoglobulin deposits and complementary components along the dermoepidermal junction in LE patients. LBT can be helpful in differentiation between SLE systemic lupus erythematosus (SLE) and CCLE. In SLE patients LBT is often positive in both unaffected and affected skin, whereas in CCLE patients only the affected skin is positive [6]. In LPP, DIF patterns consist of numerous globular deposits of immunoglobulins, particularly IgM (colloid bodies), and deposits of C3 in the papillary dermis [13, 14]. There are studies showing that immuno reactants (C3, IgG and IgM) may be present across the basement membrane in polymorphous light eruptions. However, when accumulation is present, it is generally weak [4].

Interpretation of skin biopsy material in connective tissue diseases is performed together with serological status, clinical presentation and immunofluorescence studies. The dermatopathologist can play an important role in the diagnosis, proper classification, prognosis, and treatment of a patient with connective tissue disease.

Based on the clinical picture, DIF and histology, the presented patient was diagnosed with DLE.

Key Points
- The most common form of chronic cutaneous lupus erythematosus is discoid lupus erythematosus
- Scalp involvement of DLE can cause scaring alopecia

References

1. McDaniel B, Sukumaran S, Tanner LS. Discoid lupus erythematosus. [Updated 2020 Aug 15]. In: StatPearls [internet]. Treasure Island (FL): StatPearls Publishing; 2020. Available from: https://www.ncbi.nlm.nih.gov/books/NBK493145/.
2. Gaüzère L, Gerber A, Renou F, Ferrandiz D, Bagny K, Osdoit S, Yvin JL, Raffray L. Epidemiology of systemic lupus erythematosus in Reunion Island, Indian Ocean: a case-series in adult patients from a university hospital. Rev Med Interne. 2019 Apr;40(4):214–9.
3. Kuhn A. Cutaneous manifestations of lupus erythematosus. Handbook Syst Autoimmun Dis. 2006;5:49–59.
4. McKee PH. McKee's pathology of the skin. 4th ed. Edinburgh: Elsevier/Saunders; 2012.
5. Kuhn A, Lehmann P, Ruzicka T, editors. Cutaneous lupus erythematosus. Dusseldorf: Springer; 2005.
6. Patterson JW, editor. Weedon's skin pathology. 4th ed. Elsevier Limited; 2016.
7. Saleh D, Crane JS. Tumid Lupus Erythematosus. In: StatPearls [Internet]. Treasure Island (FL): StatPearls Publishing; 2020 Aug 16.
8. Guarrera M. Polymorphous light eruption. Ultraviolet light in human health. Diseases and Environment. 2017:61–70.
9. Reich A, Marcinow K, Bialynicki-Birula R. The lupus band test in systemic lupus erythematosus patients. Ther Clin Risk Manag. 2011;7:27–32.
10. Bunagan MJK, Banka N, Shapiro J. Hair loss in lupus erythematosus. In: Encyclopedia of medical immunology–autoimmune diseases. New York: Springer Science + Business Media; 2014. p. 455–9.
11. Chung HJ, Goldberg LJ. Histologic features of chronic cutaneous lupus erythematosus of the scalp using horizontal sectioning: emphasis on follicular findings. J Am Acad Dermatol. 2017;77:349–55.
12. Rongioletti F, Christana K. Cicatricial (scarring) alopecias. Am J Clin Dermatol. 2012;13:247–60.
13. Trachsler S, Trueb RM. Value of direct immunofluorescence for differential diagnosis of cicatricial alopecia. Dermatology. 2005;211:98–102.
14. Donati A, Gupta AK, Jacob C, Cavelier-Balloy B, Reygagne P. The use of direct immunofluorescence in frontal Fibrosing alopecia. Skin Appendage Disord. 2017;3(3):125–8.

Chapter 16
A Difficult Case of Alopecia

Satya Wydya Yenny, Sigya Octari, and Rahma Ledika Veroci

A 23-year-old Indonesian man presented with hairless patches on the scalp which has increased in size and number since one month (Fig. 16.1). No itching, redness or dandruff were reported. There was no history of long-term medications, malignancy, hair pulling, chemotherapy, injected drug usage. No history of hair loss in his family was reported.

On physical examination, coin-shaped areas of non-scarring hair loss were observed. A hair pull test was negative. A trichoscopic examination revealed exclamation mark hair, cadaver hairs (black dots), and yellow dots (Fig. 16.1). Fungal culture as well as syphilis serology and antinuclear antibodies tests were negative. Thyroid function tests were normal. A micronutrient investigation showed zinc deficiency (59 ug/dl).

Based on the case description and the photographs, what is the most likely diagnosis?

1. Alopecia areata.
2. Latent syphilis.
3. Tinea capitis.

S. W. Yenny (✉) · S. Octari · R. L. Veroci
Department of Dermatology and Venereology, Cosmetic Dermatology Division, Universitas Andalas, Padang, Indonesia

Faculty of Medicine, Universitas Andalas, Padang, Indonesia

Dr. M. Djamil Hospital, Padang, Indonesia

Indonesian Society of Dermatology and Venereology, Jakarta, Indonesia
e-mail: satyawidyayenny@med.unand.ac.id

A. Waśkiel-Burnat et al. (eds.), *Clinical Cases in Hair Disorders*, Clinical Cases in Dermatology, https://doi.org/10.1007/978-3-030-93423-1_16

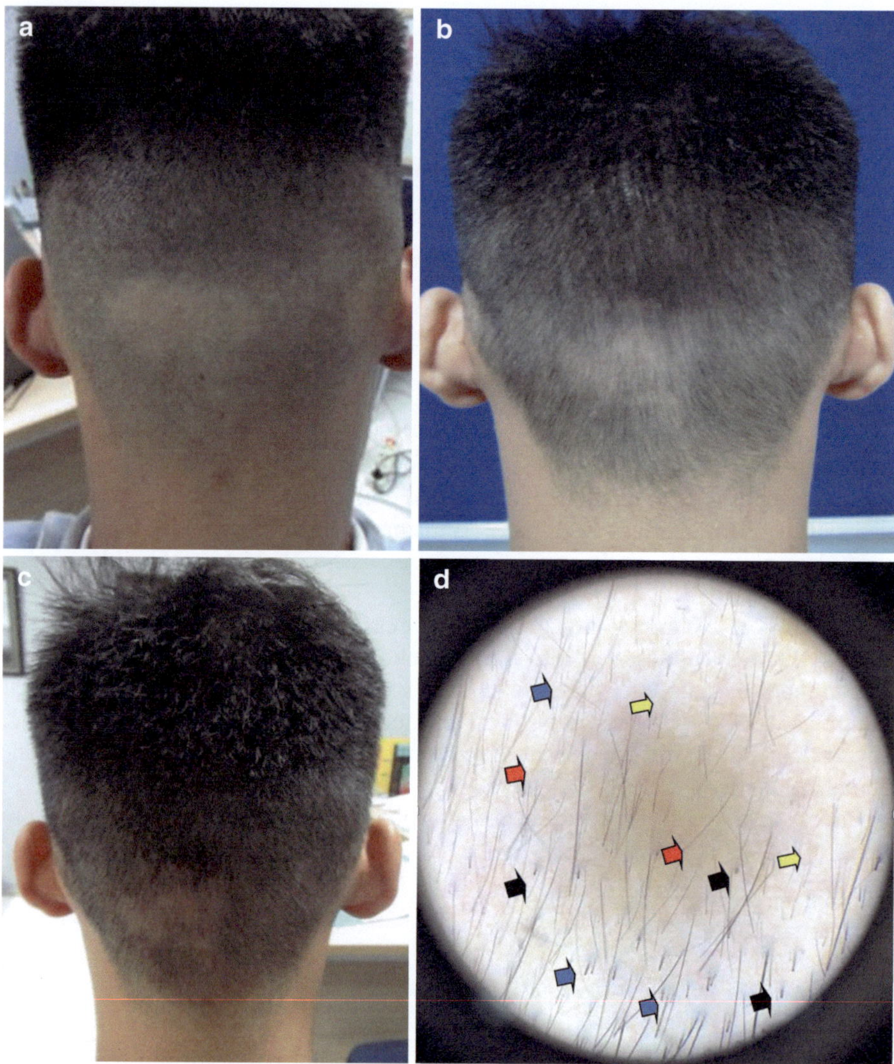

Fig. 16.1 A 23-year-old man with hair loss. (**a**) Before treatment. (**b**, **c**) After treatment. (**d**) Trichoscopy shows exclamation mark hair (red arrow), yellow dot (yellow arrow), broken hair (blue arrow) and black dots (black arrow)

Diagnosis

Alopecia areata.

Discussion

Alopecia areata (AA) is characterized by an acute onset. It typically presents as oval or round, well-circumscribed, hairless patches with a smooth surface. Characteristic hallmarks of alopecia areata are black dots that result from hair that breaks off by the time it reaches the skin surface. Exclamation mark hairs which have a thicker distal end and taper proximally, appear when the broken hairs are pushed out of the hair follicle. Alopecia areata usually is asymptomatic but it may cause mild itching and erythema. Nail involvement may occur with pitting or sandpaper-like appearance [1].

Alopecia areata may be associated with thyroid disease, syphilis, micronutrients deficiency, systemic lupus erythematosus and hereditary syndromes [1, 2].

Zinc is a micro nutrient that is involved in protein function, cell signaling, and gene expression. Zinc is also important for a function and proper immune cell response. As an essential element, zinc must be supplied to the human body through food. One of the symptoms of a severe zinc deficiency is alopecia [3].

Zinc is required for functional activity of hair follicles and helps in hair follicle recovery. It comes out of the oil attached to the hair follicles which keeps the sebum and prevents dryness of the hair. Zinc deficiency actually causes damage of the protein structure of hair follicles. This weakness of hair follicles leads to hair loss. Zinc deficiency interferes with the production of DNA and RNA needed for normal hair follicle cell division and the developmental stage of hair growth [4].

Superpotent (class I) and potent (class II) topical corticosteroids are widely used to treat alopecia areata [5]. During treatment, zinc levels must be monitored because overdose of corticosteroids may lead to copper or calcium deficiency, drowsiness, and headaches. The recommended daily amount of zinc for men and pregnant women is 11 mg and for women is 8 mg. In zinc deficiency, the recommended daily dose for adults is 25 up to 50 mg elemental zinc, while for children 0.5 to 1 mg/kg [6]. The presented patient was diagnosed with alopecia areata coexisted with zinc deficiency. Clobetasole propionate 0.05% cream in occlusion applied twice daily and zinc tablet 40 mg daily were recommended. A significant improvement was seen after eight weeks.

Key Points
- Alopecia areata is the most common form of patchy hair loss, which is caused by immune-mediated attack of the hair follicle
- The etiology and exact pathogenesis of alopecia areata are still not well understood. The role of micronutrients deficiency has been suggested

References

1. Alkhalifah A. Alopecia areata update. Dermatol Clin. 2013;31(1):93–108.
2. Bhavani V, Devi NP. Signs are brisk when nutrients are at risk, act fast before last!!': A study on impact of nutritional intake on clinical manifestation. Galore Int J Health Sci Res. 2020;5(1):20–7.
3. Madeline J, Bedford LM, Potts GA. Clinical efficacy of popular oral hair growth supplement ingredients. Int J Dermatol. 2020;1-12
4. Rahman F, Akter QS. Serum zinc and copper levels in alopecia. J-Bangladesh Soc Physiol. 2019;14(1):21–5.
5. Otberg N, Saphiro J. Alopecia Areata. In: Kang S, Amagam M, Brucker A, Enk AH, Margolis David J, Mcmichael AJ, et al., editors. Fitzpatrick's dermatology in general medicine. 9th ed. USA: McGraw-Hill Companies; 2019. p. 1517–22.
6. Andreas M, Finner. Nutrition and hair deficiencies and supplements. Dermatol Clin. 2013;31:167–72.

Chapter 17
A Man with Alopecia, Abnormal Nails, and Thickened Plantar Skin

Cleo Rochat, Hannah Singer, George Kroumpouzos, and John Kawaoka

A 58-year-old man of French-Canadian ancestry presented with thinning hair, thick skin on the soles, and abnormal fingernails and toenails. At birth he was noted to have thin white hair on his scalp and abnormal fingernails. Since childhood, he reported having thin nails that would break easily and thin hair with sparse eyebrows and eyelashes. He had kept his head shaved for the last 20 years. He reported the soles of his feet had thickened, yellow skin which also started in childhood and had become progressively worse with age. His medical history was otherwise notable for melanoma of the right leg, basal cell carcinoma of the forehead, and eczema. His father and paternal grandmother had similar abnormal nails and sparse hair. He denied any pain in the nail or digits, any dental abnormalities, visual impairment, abnormal sweating or photophobia.

On exam he was well appearing with diffuse alopecia, absent eyebrows and eyelashes, and sparse body hair. All twenty fingernails and toenails were absent or short with dystrophic, thickened nail plates with rough edges. Bilateral weight bearing

C. Rochat
Warren Alpert Medical School of Brown University, Providence, RI, USA
e-mail: Cleo_Rochat@brown.edu

H. Singer · J. Kawaoka (✉)
Warren Alpert Medical School of Brown University, Providence, RI, USA

Brown Dermatology, Inc., Providence, RI, USA
e-mail: Hannah_Singer@brown.edu; John_Kawaoka@brown.edu

G. Kroumpouzos
Warren Alpert Medical School of Brown University, Providence, RI, USA

GK Dermatology, South Weymouth, MA, USA

Department of Dermatology, Medical School of Jundiaí, São Paulo, Brazil
e-mail: George.Kroumpouzos@GKderm.com

A. Waśkiel-Burnat et al. (eds.), *Clinical Cases in Hair Disorders*, Clinical Cases in Dermatology, https://doi.org/10.1007/978-3-030-93423-1_17

areas of palmar feet had hyperkeratotic yellow plaques. There were no oral mucosal or dental abnormalities.

Based on the case description and photographs, what is your diagnosis?

Differential Diagnoses

1. Hidrotic ectodermal dysplasia (Clouston syndrome).
2. Hypohidrotic ectodermal dysplasia (Christ-Siemens-Touraine syndrome).
3. Pachyonychia congenita.

Diagnosis

Hidrotic ectodermal dysplasia (Clouston syndrome).

Discussion

Clouston syndrome, or hidrotic ectodermal dysplasia, is an autosomal dominant disorder that typically presents with a triad of dystrophic nails, hypotrichosis or alopecia, and palmoplantar hyperkeratosis. Hidrotic ectodermal dysplasia is a subtype of ectodermal dysplasia, which is a larger group of disorders marked by abnormal embryogenesis of ectodermal tissue such as hair, sweat glands, nails, teeth, and sebaceous glands. There are many variants of ectodermal dysplasias, including hypohidrotic and hidrotic subtypes [1].

Mutations in the *GJB6* gene, located on chromosome 13, are implicated in the pathogenesis of Clouston syndrome. *GJB6* encodes the connexin 30 protein, found in gap junctions between adjacent cells. There are several *GJB6* mutations that have been reported in the pathogenesis of Clouston syndrome, as well as a report of a sporadic case of hidrotic ectodermal dysplasia without a *GJB6* mutation [2, 3]. Clouston syndrome displays an autosomal dominant inheritance pattern with likely 100% penetrance [2]. This patient noted his father and maternal grandfather had Clouston syndrome as well, but the patient's siblings were unaffected. The patient in this case has no children and did not desire genetic testing, but genetic counseling should be offered to all patients with suspected inherited disorders that may affect their family planning.

Clinical features that are highly suggestive of Clouston syndrome include nail abnormalities, palmoplantar keratoderma, and alopecia. Dystrophic nails may initially appear milky white in childhood, and progress into short and thickened or triangular shaped nails with distal separation from the nail plate. Hyperkeratosis can

Fig. 17.1 Diffuse alopecia and hypotrichosis of the face. An incidental bruise is noted on left cheek

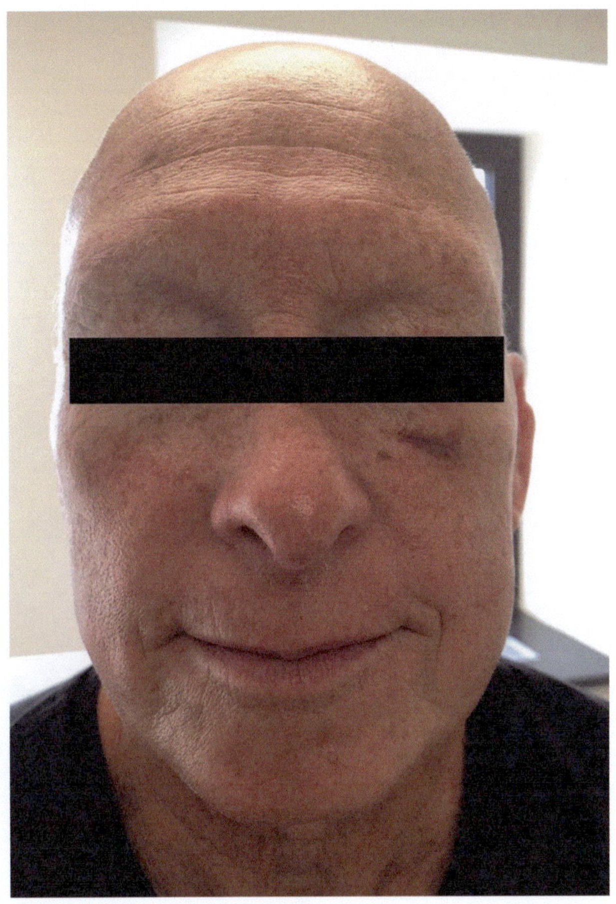

be seen on the surface of the palms and soles, which is progressive with age. Alopecia in Clouston syndrome manifests with either progressive partial or total hair loss, most often affecting the eyebrows, lashes, axillary and pubic hair [1, 2]. Eccrine sweat glands and dentition are normal in Clouston syndrome, which is a point of differentiation from hypohidrotic ectodermal dysplasia, or Christ-Siemens-Touraine syndrome. Pachyonychia congenita is associated with keratin mutations and has prominent nail findings without hypotrichosis or alopecia [2].

If biopsy of affected skin is performed, the histologic findings in Clouston syndrome include orthohyperkeratosis with a normal granular layer, decreased hair shaft cuticles, and disorganized follicles [1]. Clouston syndrome can be diagnosed clinically and, if desired, confirmed with genetic testing (Figs. 17.1, 17.2, and 17.3).

The management for individuals with Clouston syndrome involves treatment of bothersome symptoms. For nail dystrophy, artificial nails may be helpful and nail

Fig. 17.2 Thickened, ragged, and absent fingernails (**a** & **b**) and toenails (**c**)

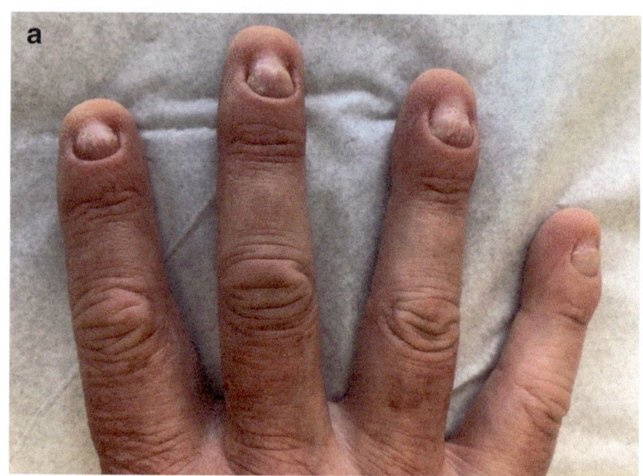

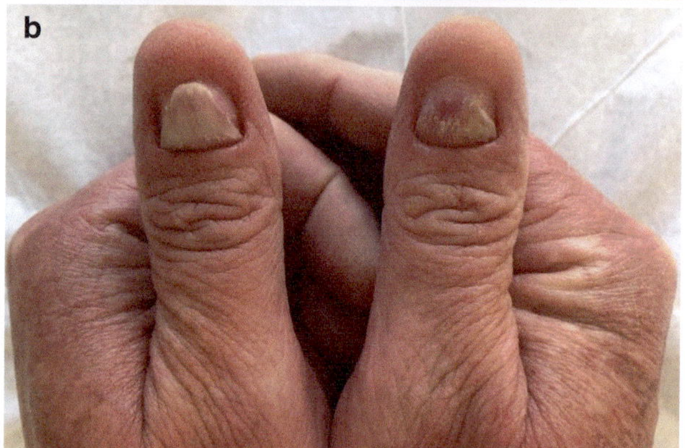

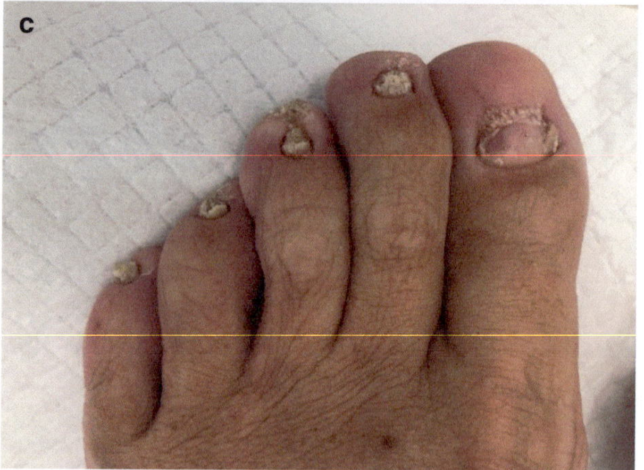

Fig. 17.3 Diffuse, yellowish, hyperkeratotic plaques are shown on the sole of right foot

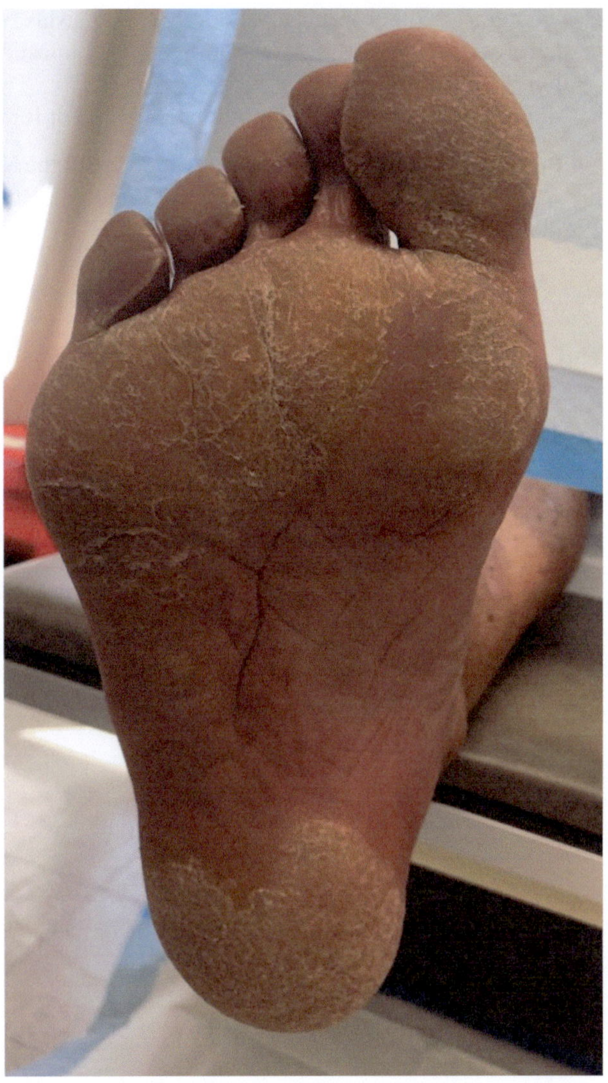

matrix ablation is an option for pain management. For alopecia, a report of a patient with Clouston syndrome found improved hair growth from treatment with topical minoxidil and tretinoin [4]. Topical emollients, keratolytics, and filing of hardened skin can be helpful for palmoplantar hyperkeratosis [2].

Key Points
- Clouston syndrome is an autosomal dominant disorder caused GJB6 mutations which lead to abnormal connexin 30 protein in gap junctions and is diagnosed based on clinical features with genetic testing available for confirmation and family planning

- In contrast to other forms of ectodermal dysplasias such as hypohidrotic ectodermal dysplasia, Clouston syndrome displays normal eccrine sweat gland functioning and dentition
- Management is based on symptomatic treatment for affected skin, hair, and nails

Comment This case was presented at a meeting of the New England Dermatological Society at the Warren Alpert Medical School of Brown University on October 17, 2020.

References

1. Metze D, Oji V. Palmoplantar keratodermas. In: Bolognia JL, Schaffer JV, Cerroni L, editors. Dermatology. Edinburgh: Elsevier; 2018. p. 924–43.
2. Mellerio J, Greenblatt D. Hidrotic ectodermal dysplasia 2. In: Adam MP, Ardinger HH, Pagon RA, et al., editors. GeneReviews® [Internet]. Seattle (WA): University of Washington, Seattle; 2005. 1993–2021. Available at https://www.ncbi.nlm.nih.gov/books/NBK1200.
3. Nakamura M, Ishikawa O. A patient with alopecia, nail dystrophy, palmoplantar hyperkeratosis, keratitis, hearing difficulty and micrognathia without GJB2 or GJB6 mutations: a new type of hidrotic ectodermal dysplasia? Br J Dermatol. 2007;156:777–9.
4. Melkote S, Dhurat RS, Palav A, Jerajani HR. Alopecia in congenital hidrotic ectodermal dysplasia responding to treatment with a combination of topical minoxidil and tretinoin. Int J Dermatol. 2009;48:184–5.

Chapter 18
Alopecia in a Linear Pattern

Zekayi Kutlubay, Defne Özkoca, and Server Serdaroğlu

A four-year-old boy, with coexisted linear and whorled nevoid hypermelanosis and inflammatory linear verrucous epidermal nevus on the left lower extremity, presented with a recurrent patchy hair loss since he was three months old. He was previously treated with minoxidil 5% solution for one and a half years. Hair growth was observed; however, hair loss recurred after the drug was discontinued. His past medical history and family history were unremarkable. Laboratory work-up including the vitamins and minerals were normal for the age.

A physical examination revealed linear patchy alopecia on the scalp (Fig. 18.1). Moreover, generalized hyperpigmented linear and whorled streaks with sharp midline demarcation on the left lower extremity as well as the left side of the abdomen and chest (Figs. 18.2 and 18.3) were observed. The hyperpigmented lesion on the left lower extremity had a verrucous surface (Fig. 18.4). On the posterior neck a linear, whorled hypopigmented patch was present (Fig. 18.5). Trichoscopy showed exclamation mark hairs, broken hairs, regrowing hairs of different length, yellow and black dots.

Histology showed 20 terminal hair follicles and 16 vellus hair follicles. There were seven vellus and seven terminal anagen stage hair follicles; nine vellus and 13 terminal catagen and telogen stage hair follicles. No follicular stellae were present. Mild spongiosis and exocytosis were observed around the hair follicles.

Based on the case description and the photographs, what is your diagnosis for the hair disease?

1. Alopecia areata.
2. Lupus erythematous profundus.

Z. Kutlubay (✉) · D. Özkoca · S. Serdaroğlu
Cerrahpaşa Medical Faculty, Department of Dermatology, İstanbul University-Cerrahpaşa, Istanbul, Turkey

A. Waśkiel-Burnat et al. (eds.), *Clinical Cases in Hair Disorders*, Clinical Cases in Dermatology, https://doi.org/10.1007/978-3-030-93423-1_18

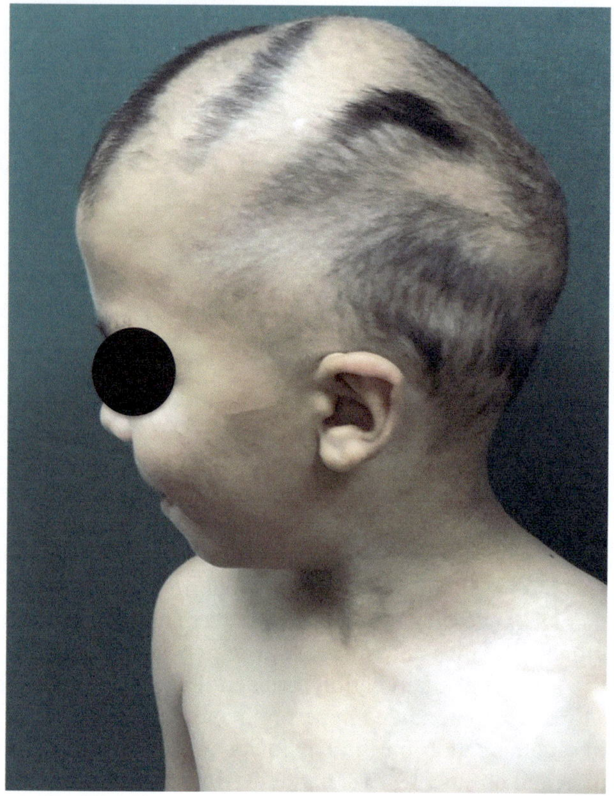

Fig. 18.1 Linear patchy alopecia on the scalp

Diagnosis

Alopecia areata.

Discussion

Alopecia areata is a common type of hair loss that presents with inflammatory, non-scarring and well-demarcated alopecic patches. It is seen in approximately 0.2% of the population. The disease is seen equally in both sexes and all ages groups can be affected. Alopecia areata has an autoimmune pathogenesis: the immune privileged state of the anagen hairs is disturbed; and as a result, dystrophic hair cycling with a premature entrance to the telogen state is observed. Due to its autoimmune nature, alopecia areata is more prevalent in patients with other autoimmune diseases. Furthermore, it is more common in patients with the atopic diathesis. Nail changes

Fig. 18.2 Generalized hyperpigmented linear and whorled streaks on the left side of the abdomen and chest

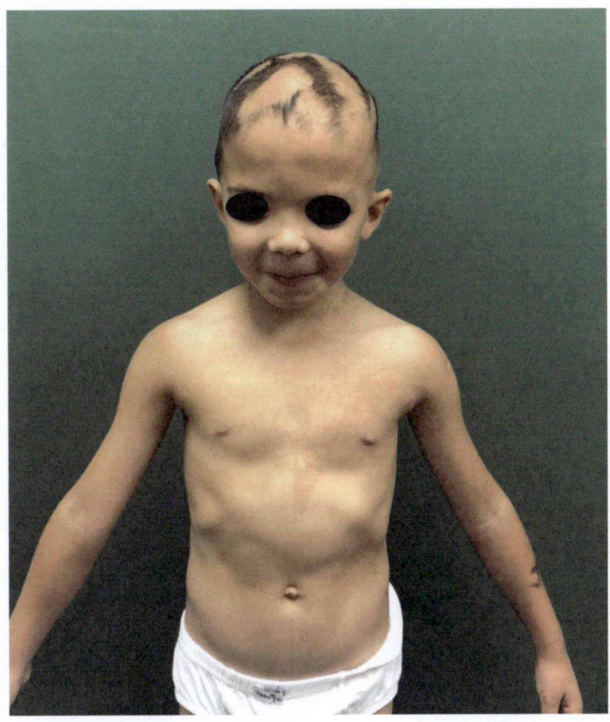

such as pitting, brittleness and striations are seen in up to 20% of the patients with alopecia areata. Trichoscopy is helpful in the diagnosis of the disease. Dystrophic hairs, exclamation point hairs, black dots and yellow dots are characteristic trichoscopic features. In an acute phase of alopecia areata, histopathology reveals peribulbar lymphocytic inflammation (both CD4 and CD8) and an increased number of catagen and telogen hairs. In chronic lesions there is the lack of peribulbar inflammation but miniaturization is present. Although the hair loss is reversible in nature, prognosis is poor in the patients with younger age of the disease onset or the ophiasis subtype [1]. Treatment modalities are chosen according to the duration of the diseases, extent of the disease and the patient's age. Intralesional corticosteroids are the mainstay of treatment. Topical corticosteroids can be used if intralesional steroids are contraindicated or not available. Systemic therapy is indicated in patients with severe disease who are older than 13 years. The systemic treatment options are corticosteroids, cyclosporine, methotrexate and jannus-kinase inhibitors [2]. Topical immunotherapy or anthralin can be used in recalcitrant cases as well [3].

There are previous reports of alopecia areata with a linear presentation, all of which were misdiagnosed as non-scarring alopecia caused by lupus erythematosus profundus initially. Dermoscopy and histopathology can be used to differentiate

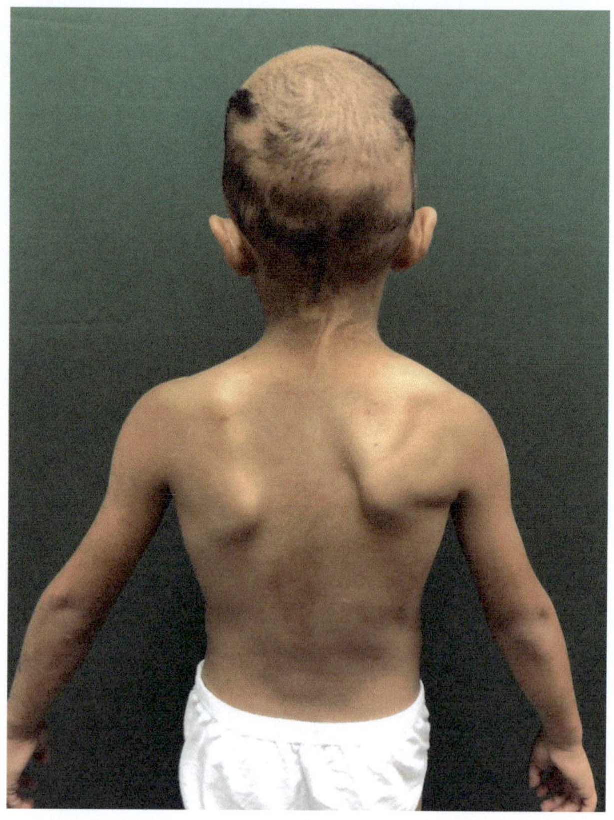

Fig. 18.3 Generalized hyperpigmented linear and whorled streaks on the left side of the trunk

these two diseases. Alopecia areata is characterized by a decreased ratio of anagen to catagen and telogen hair follicles; an increased number of vellus follicles; and a "swarm of bees-like" lymphocytic inflammation around the hair follicles. On the contrary, lupus erythematous profundus demonstrates lobular lymphohistiocytic infliltrate with plasma cells in the adipose tissue along with stromal mucin deposition [4, 5].

The presented patient was diagnosed with alopecia areata. Topical corticosteroid preparation (once a day) was prescribed to the patchy areas. The patient is still on therapy; partial hair regrowth is observed.

Fig. 18.4 Inflammatory linear verrucous epidermal nevus on the left lower extremity

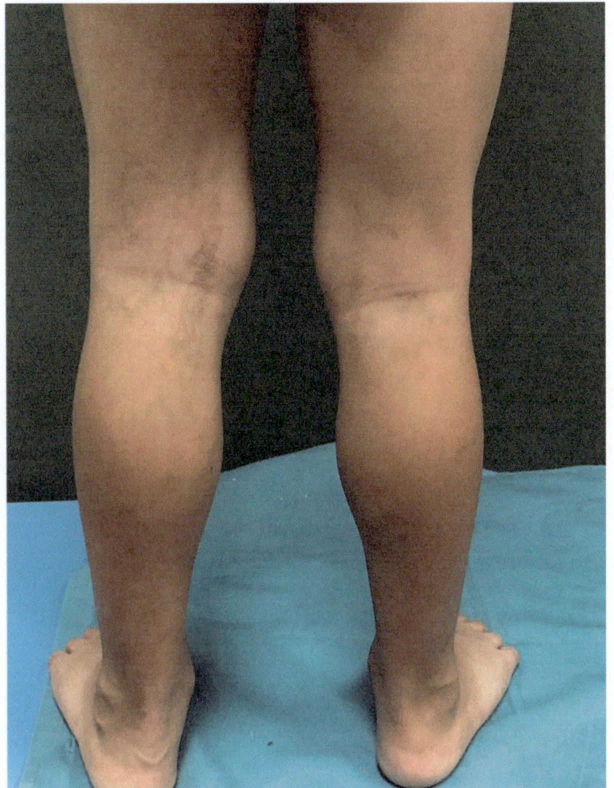

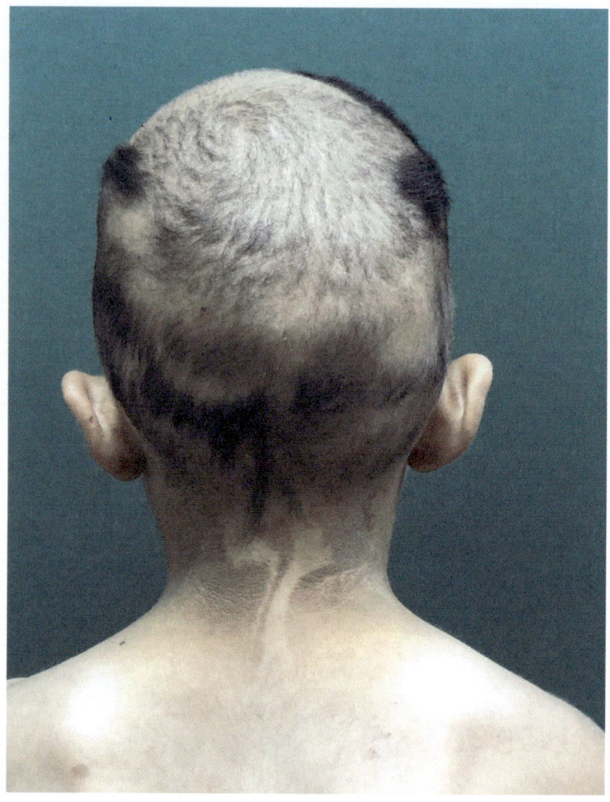

Fig. 18.5 The posterior neck with a linear, whorled hypopigmented patch

Key Points

- Alopecia areata is a common type of hair loss that presents as non-scarring and well-demarcated hairless areas
- Trichoscopy shows dystrophic hairs, exclamation point hairs, black dots and yellow dots
- In acute alopecia areata, peribulbar lymphocytic inflammation (both CD4 and CD8) and an increased number of catagen and telogen hairs are observed. In chronic lesions there is the lack the peribulbar inflammation but miniaturization is present
- Linear alopecia areata can be misdiagnosed as lupus erythematosus profundus. Dermoscopy and histopathology can be used to differentiate these two diseases

References

1. Strazzulla LC, Wang EHC, Avila L, Lo Sicco K, Brinster N, Christiano AM, Shapiro J. Alopecia areata: disease characteristics, clinical evaluation, and new perspectives on pathogenesis. J Am Acad Dermatol. 2018;78(1):1–12. https://doi.org/10.1016/j.jaad.2017.04.1141.

2. Meah N, Wall D, York K, Bhoyrul B, Bokhari L, Sigall DA, Bergfeld WF, Betz RC, Blume-Peytavi U, Callender V, Chitreddy V, Combalia A, Cotsarelis G, Craiglow B, Donovan J, Eisman S, Farrant P, Green J, Grimalt R, Harries M, Hordinsky M, Irvine AD, Itami S, Jolliffe V, King B, Lee WS, McMichael A, Messenger A, Mirmirani P, Olsen E, Orlow SJ, Piraccini BM, Rakowska A, Reygagne P, Roberts JL, Rudnicka L, Shapiro J, Sharma P, Tosti A, Vogt A, Wade M, Yip L, Zlotogorski A, Sinclair R. The alopecia Areata consensus of experts (ACE) study: results of an international expert opinion on treatments for alopecia areata. J Am Acad Dermatol. 2020;83(1):123–30. https://doi.org/10.1016/j.jaad.2020.03.004.
3. Kagami S, Kishi Y, Hino H. Topical immunotherapy in combination with anthralin in the treatment of refractory alopecia areata. J Cosmet Dermatol. 2020;19(9):2411–4. https://doi.org/10.1111/jocd.13588.
4. Shetty S, Rao R, Kudva RR, Subramanian K. Linear alopecia areata. Int J Trichol. 2016;8(3):144–5. https://doi.org/10.4103/0974-7753.189017.
5. Yu L, Lu Z. Linear alopecia areata. JAAD Case Rep. 2018;4(10):1072–3. https://doi.org/10.1016/j.jdcr.2018.08.015.

Chapter 19
An Elderly Female with Alopecia

Mao Lu, Yu-Ping Ran, Ya-Ling Dai, Kai-Wen Zhuang, Sushmita Pradhan, and Wen-Ying Hu

A 57-year-old woman presented with an one-year history of an itchy area of hair loss on the vertex. She also reported diffuse hair loss on the frontoparietal area of the scalp since 10 years. Her granddaughter, who she took care of, had similar patchy alopecia since three months.

A physical examination revealed diffuse hair loss on the frontoparietal area and patchy hair loss with the presence of black dots on the vertex region (Fig. 19.1a).

Based on the case description and the photograph, what is your diagnosis of the grandma?

1. Androgenetic alopecia.
2. Tinea capitis.

Diagnosis

Tinea capitis with seborrheic alopecia.

M. Lu
Department of Dermatovenereology, West China Hospital, Sichuan University, Chengdu, China

Department of Dermatovenereology, The First Affiliated Hospital of Chengdu Medical College, Chengdu, China

Y.-P. Ran (✉) · K.-W. Zhuang · S. Pradhan · W.-Y. Hu
Department of Dermatovenereology, West China Hospital, Sichuan University, Chengdu, China

Y.-L. Dai
Department of Laboratory Medicine, West China Hospital, Sichuan University, Chengdu, China

A. Waśkiel-Burnat et al. (eds.), *Clinical Cases in Hair Disorders*, Clinical Cases in Dermatology, https://doi.org/10.1007/978-3-030-93423-1_19

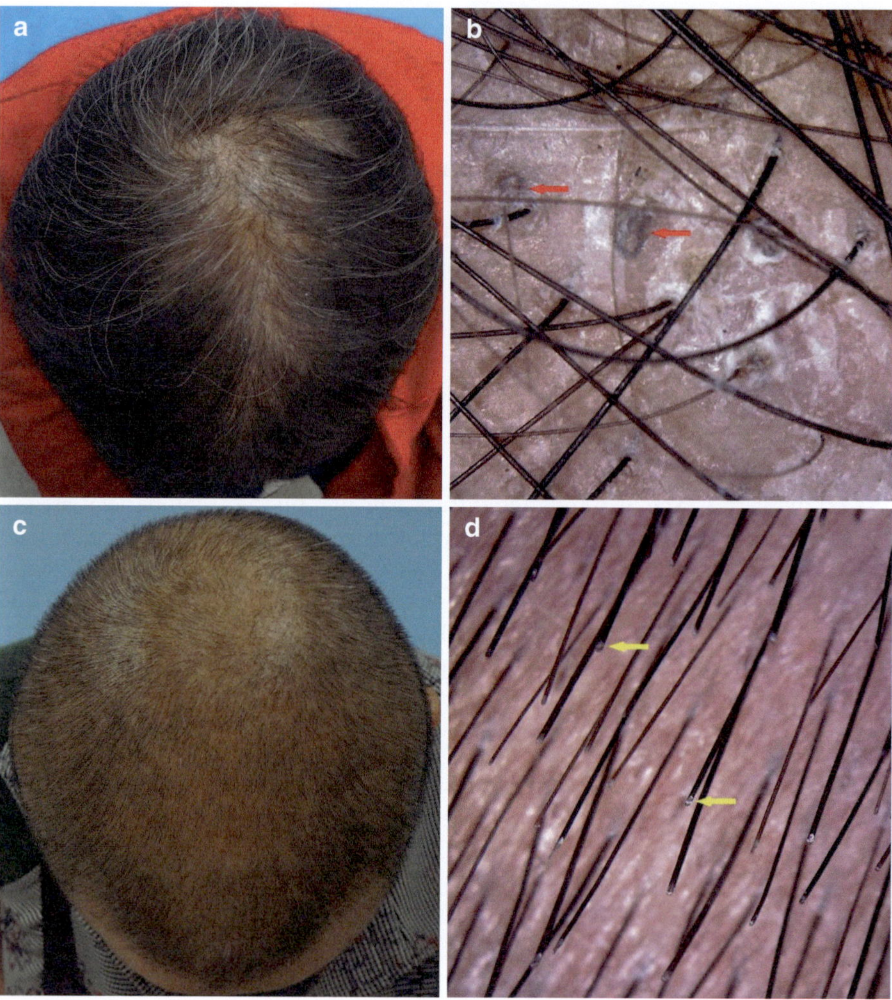

Fig. 19.1 (a) A 57-year-old woman with diffuse hair loss on the frontoparietal area and patchy hair loss on the vertex region. (b) Dermoscopy shows corkscrew hairs (red arrows) covered by scales (×25). (c) Clinical picture after therapy. (d) Follow-up dermoscopy shows cigarette-ash-shaped hairs (yellow arrows) (×25)

In the presented patient dermoscopy showed numerous short, highly convoluted, coiled and twisted corkscrew hairs (Fig. 19.1b). A direct mycological examination, in woman and her granddaughter, showed curved hairs fully filled with extremely high numbers of endothrix spores (Fig. 19.2a, b). Cultures inoculated with samples from two patients on Sabouraud glucose agar slants after incubation at 28 °C for seven days both yielded floccose and faint yellow colonies (Fig. 19.2c). A microscopic examination of slide cultures with lactophenol cotton blue stain showed irregular branching hyphae with septa in various diameter and numerous akinetes

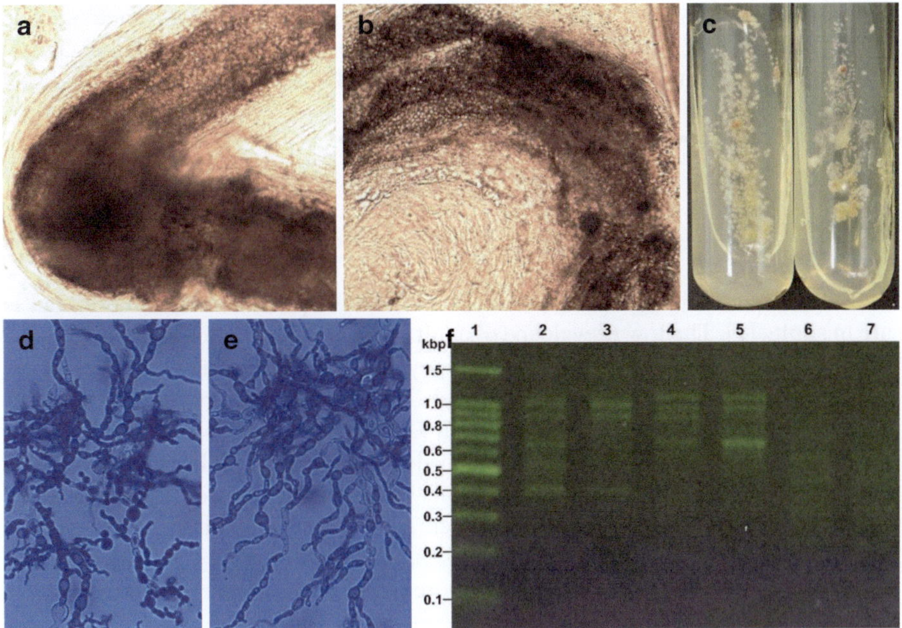

Fig. 19.2 A direct mycological examination with potassium hydroxide in child (**a**) and woman (**b**) Curved hairs fully filled with extremely high numbers of endothrix spores (×400) (**c**) Cultures inoculated with samples from child (left) and woman (right) yield floccose and faint yellow colonies. Slide-culture of *Trichophyton violaceum* from child (**d**) and woman (**e**) reveals irregular branching hyphae with septa in various diameter and numerous akinetes (lactophenol cotton-blue staining, ×400) (**f**) RAPD band patterns of the two isolates. Lane 1, size marker; 2, OPAO-15 (girl); 3, OPAO-15 (the woman); 4, ATG (girl); 5, ATG (woman); 6, ATGS (girl); 7, ATGS (woman)

(Fig. 19.2d, e). Fungal DNA samples were amplified with the microsatellite primers (T1.forward 5′-GTA AGG ATG GCT AGT TAG GGG, T1.reverse 5′-TGG TCT GGC CTT GAC TGA CC). The sequences were aligned (BIOEDIT, http://www. mbio.ncsu.edu/) and deposited in the GenBank with the accession number KP339818 (isolated from the girl, 227 bp) and KP339819 (isolated from the woman, 232 bp). The two DNA sequences of the isolated fungi were in accordance with *Trichophyton violaceum* (DDBJ/EMBL/GenBank accession No. AJ745082.1) with the homology of 98% and 99% by using the Blast 2 Sequences Tool (http://www. ncbi.nlm.nih.gov/blast/bl2seq/wblast2.cgi). Primers ATGS [5'-ATGGATC(G,C) (G,C)C-3'], ATG (5'-ATGGATCGGC-3′), and OPAO-15 (5'-GAAGGCTCCC-3′) were used for random amplified polymorphic DNA (RAPD) analysis. The two *Trichophyton violaceum* isolates showed distinct and similar band patterns, which suggested that they might have come from the same source (Fig. 19.2f).

Based on the morphological features and molecular identification, the patient was diagnosed with tinea capitis (black-dot ringworm) and alopecia seborrheica. She received systemic treatment with itraconazole (400 mg a day) and topical treatment with 1% naftifine-0.25% ketoconazole cream after wash of 2% ketoconazole shampoo once a day. She was cured after six weeks of treatment without any side effect (Fig. 19.1c). Post-treatment dermoscopy revealed a number of cigarette-ash-shapped hairs and long normal hair (Fig. 19.1d). No recurrence was observed after six months follow-up.

Discussion

Tinea capitis is a common fungal infection of the scalp and hair in children but is rare in adults [1]. The low prevalence of adult tinea capitis could be explained by the relative resistance of adult hair to dermatophytes colonization due to the fungistatic properties of saturated long-chain fatty acids in the sebum. Most of adult tinea capitis cases occur in post-menopausal women [2]. This occurrence is probably due to the reduction of sebaceous secretion and decreased fungicidal properties of the sebum [2, 3]. Tinea capitis in adults presents with variable degrees of inflammatory reactions: from glabrous type, to seborrheic dermatitis-like pattern, to 'black-dot' pattern, to discoid lupus erythematosus-resembling lesion, to grey patches to kerion [4, 5]. The noninflammatory lesions are more common than the inflammatory ones. The seborrheic dermatitis type and the glabrous type of tinea capitis are common in adults but kerion and grey patches are rare [4]. Adult tinea capitis may show polymorphic and atypical clinical presentations leading to difficulty in diagnosis and delay in treatment. The erroneous notion of the disease being uncommon and the frequent atypical clinical presentation requires a high degree of clinical suspicion. Recent studies have reported that some dermoscopic features of infected hairs may be valuable for the diagnosis of tinea capitis, such as comma hairs and corkscrew hairs. These findings may become of value for diagnosing tinea capitis and be used for easy and inexpensive treatment monitoring in tinea capitis. The presented patient was initially diagnosed with isolated alopecia seborrheica. However, tinea capitis was suggested by the presence of corkscrew hairs in the 'black-dot' area of the scalp. By further mycological examination, the diagnosis of tinea capitis caused by *Trichophyton violaceum* was confirmed.

Adult tinea capitis is usually acquired via hairdressing equipment or in childcare settings. Other possible explanations include extensions of an infection from glabrous skin or nails [1]. In the present cases, RAPD analysis indicated two isolates was the same strain. We therefore speculate that the shared items between the girl and her grandma, such as the comb, pillow or towel, might be the vector of the dermatophytic infection.

Key Points
- Most of adult tinea capitis cases occur in post-menopausal women due to the reduction of sebaceous secretion and decreased fungicidal properties of the sebum
- Dermoscopy may be used as a fast, noninvasive, reliable and inexpensive method for the diagnosis of tinea capitis

References

1. Yu J, et al. Current topics of tinea capitis in China. Nippon Ishinkin Gakkai Zasshi. 2005;46(2):61–6.
2. Cremer G, et al. Tinea capitis in adults: misdiagnosis or reappearance? Dermatology. 1997;194(1):8–11.
3. Van Hecke E, et al. Tinea capitis in an adult (*Microsporum canis*). Mykosen. 1980; 23(11):607–8.
4. Kamalam A, et al. Tinea capitis an endemic disease in Madras. Mycopathologia. 1980;71(1):45–51.
5. Moberg S. Tinea capitis in the elderly. A report on two cases caused by *Trichophyton tonsurans*. Dermatologica. 1984;169(1):36–40.

Chapter 20
An Infant with Suppurative Circular Alopecia on the Scalp

Bin Yin, Yu-Ping Ran, Lixin Fu, Conghui Li, and Wenju Wang

An eight-month-old boy presented with a seven-month history of an inflammatory, suppurative, circular alopecia with diffuse scaling on his scalp (Fig. 20.1a). Six months prior to the current observations, he was diagnosed with fungal infection and treated with topical anti-fungi agents (specific information unavailable), but his condition did not improve. Before the appearance of the boy's lesion, his mother had patchy erythema and scaling on her neck. She was diagnosed with tinea corporis. The lesion was cured with topical use of terbinafine for one week. The boy was otherwise healthy without any immunosuppressive disorder and had no significant medical history.

On dermoscopic examination accumulated scales around hair roots, black dots, cigarette-ash-shaped hairs and barcode-like hairs with horizontal white bands were observed (Fig. 20.1b). Culture of secretion from the abscess was negative for bacteria. A direct mycological examination with fungal fluorescence staining showed high numbers of ectothrix spores and endothrix hyphae of the hair (Fig. 20.1c). Fungal culture inoculated from the samples of the lesions yielded woolly colonies with dense cottony surfaces and lemon-yellow pigmentation. *Arthroderma otae* (teleomorph of *Microsporum canis*) was identified by culture and sequencing of the nuclear ribosomal ITS region (No. MH401127 in GenBank).

Based on the case description and the photograph, what is your diagnosis?

B. Yin · L. Fu · C. Li · W. Wang
Department of Dermatovenereology, Chengdu Second People's Hospital, Chengdu, China

Y.-P. Ran (✉)
Department of Dermatovenereology, West China Hospital, Sichuan University, Chengdu, China

A. Waśkiel-Burnat et al. (eds.), *Clinical Cases in Hair Disorders*, Clinical Cases in Dermatology, https://doi.org/10.1007/978-3-030-93423-1_20

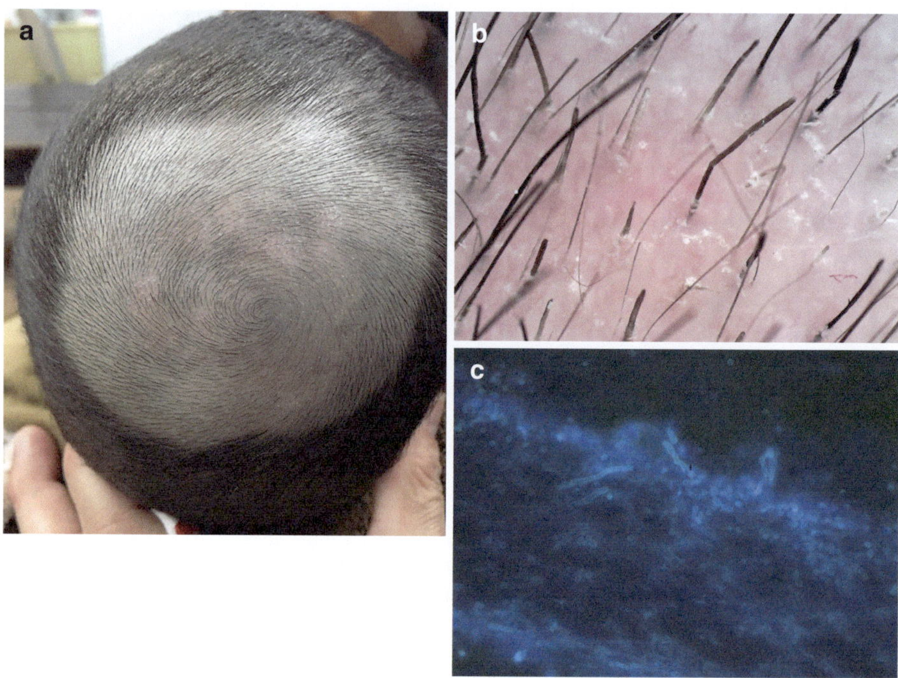

Fig. 20.1 (**a**) An eight-month-old boy presented with a seven-month history of an inflammatory suppurative circular alopecia with diffuse scaling on his scalp. (**b**) A dermoscopic examination shows accumulated scales around hair roots, black dots, cigarette-ash-shaped hairs and barcode-like hairs with horizontal white bands. (**c**) A direct mycological examination with fungal fluorescence staining shows high numbers of ectothrix spores and endothrix hyphae of the hair

Differential Diagnoses

1. Kerion.
2. Neonatal seborrheic dermatitis.
3. Carbuncle.
4. Alopecia areata.

Diagnosis

Kerion.

Discussion

Tinea capitis is an infection of scalp hair follicles and the surrounding skin, caused by dermatophyte fungi, usually species in the genera *Microsporum* and *Trichophyton*. Although less frequent than in children, tinea capitis has also been seen in infants and toddlers, even in neonates.

Different clinical presentations may arise depending on the causative organism, the type of hair invasion, and the specific host T-lymphocyte inflammatory response. In general, the zoophilic dermatophytes, typically *Microsporum canis*, are more liable to cause inflammatory responses in human, ranging from scaling erythema and/or alopecia (hair loss) to painful inflammatory masses and follicles discharging pus (kerion eruptions) [1].

An accurate diagnosis remains a vital component of management. Clinicians unfamiliar with this condition often misdiagnose tinea capitis, especially inflammatory variants such as kerions, leading to delays in diagnosis and inappropriate management. Dermoscopy is a fast, noninvasive and inexpensive method that has been recently described as useful in diagnosing tinea capitis. Characteristic trichoscopic features of tinea capitis are comma hairs, corkscrew hairs, zigzag hairs, morse code hairs and cigarette-ash-shaped hairs [2].

The presented patient was started on therapy with itraconazole oral solution (5 mg/kg/day), in addition to topical use of naftifine-ketaconazole cream daily combined with ketoconazole shampoo three times weekly. Clinical, dermoscopic and mycological examinations (light microscopy and culture) were conducted every two weeks. After four weeks of treatment with itraconazole, the inflammatory masses and scaling gradually subsided and culture was negative. Six weeks later, the lesion resolved significantly. The dermoscopic observation after complete treatment showed the cigarette-ash-shaped hairs and barcode-like hairs subsided. Oral itraconazole was continued for another two weeks. Topical therapy was stopped when the scalp scaling disappeared and hair regrowth was clinically evident. The patient was cured clinically and mycologically 70 days following treatment with no reoccurrence observed after one month of follow-up. During the course of treatment, no side effect such as dysfunction of liver and kidney was found.

Key Points
- Dermoscopy is a fast, noninvasive and inexpensive method that has been described with the specific features of tinea capitis such as comma hairs, corkscrew hairs, zigzag hairs, barcode-like hairs and cigarette-ash-shaped hairs
- The case highlights the importance of using both dermoscopy and fungal fluorescence staining, an effective and precise method, not only for facilitating the diagnosis of hair shaft infection caused by dermatophytes but also monitoring the treatment effects

References

1. Fuller LC, Barton RC, Mohd Mustapa MF, Proudfoot LE, Punjabi SP, Higgins EM. British Association of Dermatologists' guidelines for the management of tinea capitis 2014. Br J Dermatol. 2014;171(3):454–63.
2. Waskiel-Burnat A, Rakowska A, Sikora M, Ciechanowicz P, Olszewska M, Rudnicka L. Trichoscopy of Tinea Capitis: A Systematic Review. Dermatol Ther (Heidelb). 2020;10(1):43–52.

Chapter 21
Androgenetic Alopecia and Thyroid Cancer: Coincidence or More?

Uwe Wollina

A 26-year-old female patient presented with a diffuse hair loss on her scalp that developed during the last couple of years. Her medical history was remarkable for thyroid cancer eight years ago (papillary thyroid cancer T4N1M0) that was treated by thyroidectomy and subsequent radiotherapy. Thereafter, she developed hypothyreoidosis and hypoparathyroidism and was substituted with thyroxin.

Laboratory investigations showed thyroid stimulating hormone: 170 mIU/mL (normal range: 0.27–4.20), free T4: 6.32 pmol/mL (12–22), and T3: 0.63 nmol/mL (1.3–3.1).

On physical examination we observed a diffuse hair loss. The hair line did not recede (Fig. 21.1).

Based on the case description and the photographs, what is your diagnosis?

Differential Diagnoses

1. Androgenetic alopecia.
2. Alopecia areata.
3. Diffuse effluvium.
4. Paraneoplastic alopecia.
5. Radiation-induced scarring alopecia.

U. Wollina (✉)
Department of Dermatology and Allergology, Municipal Hospital of Dresden, Academic Teaching Hospital, Dresden, Germany
e-mail: Uwe.Wollina@klinikum-dresden.de

A. Waśkiel-Burnat et al. (eds.), *Clinical Cases in Hair Disorders*, Clinical Cases in Dermatology, https://doi.org/10.1007/978-3-030-93423-1_21

Fig. 21.1 A diffuse
hair loss

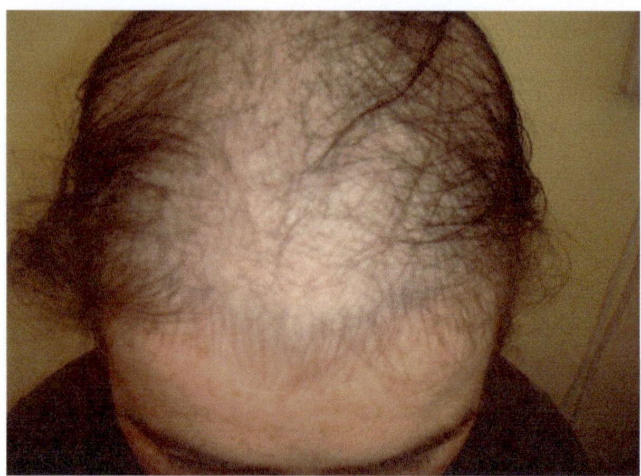

Diagnosis

Androgenetic alopecia.

Discussion

Alopecia can be divided in scarring and non-scarring types. Alopecia areata is the most common non-scarring type of hair loss. It is associated to an impairment of the immune privilege of the hair follicle. The basic pathology is perifollicular T-cell dominated inflammation. Other inflammatory non-scarring alopecia are associated with seborrheic dermatitis or psoriasis. Telogen effluvium can be related to hormonal alterations and medical drugs. Androgenetic alopecia of the female pattern differs in the micromorphology from male pattern since its more diffuse, leads seldom to complete baldness and respects the hair line. Androgenetic alopecia is more common in patients with insulin resistance, hypertension, and polycystic ovary syndrome. The hair thinning begins between puberty and 40 years of age. The inheritance pattern is polygenic. Interaction of dihydrotestosterone with androgen receptor in susceptible hair follicles activates genes which are responsible for follicular miniaturization [1].

The association between alopecia and thyroid cancer has been discussed in the literature. It was shown that a high-dose radioiodine therapy of thyroid cancer can cause a temporary alopecia in 28.1% of patients [2]. Moreover, a Taiwanese study with more than 4500 adult women confirmed that patients with alopecia had a significantly higher risk for thyroid cancer (hazard rate = 2.39, 97.5% confidence interval = 1.05–5.42) [3]. Mammalian hairless protein (HR), a 130 kDa nuclear transcription factor that is essential for proper skin and hair follicle function, may be a possible link between cancer and hair loss. HR mutations have been identified in patients with various cancers what suggest a relevance to the growth and survival of cancer cells. HR also interacts with p53 and the p53 DNA response element [4].

The presented patient was diagnosed with androgenetic alopecia.

We initiated topical treatment with 2% minoxidil [5]. There was a partial improvement after six months.

Key Points
- Androgenetic alopecia is the most common type of diffuse hair loss
- There is an association between alopecia and thyroid cancer in women
- Hair loss may also be induced by certain treatments of thyroid cancer

References

1. Martinez-Jacobo L, Villarreal-Villarreal CD, Ortiz-López R, Ocampo-Candiani J, Rojas-Martínez A. Genetic and molecular aspects of androgenetic alopecia. Indian J Dermatol Venereol Leprol. 2018;84(3):263–8.
2. Alexander C, Bader JB, Schaefer A, Finke C, Kirsch CM. Intermediate and long-term side effects of high-dose radioiodine therapy for thyroid carcinoma. J Nucl Med. 1998;39(9):1551–4.
3. Sun LM, Lin MC, Muo CH, Liang JA, Sung FC, Kao CH. Women with alopecia exhibit a higher risk for thyroid cancer: a nationwide cohort study. J Dermatol Sci. 2014;74(1):18–22.
4. Maatough A, Whitfield GK, Brook L, Hsieh D, Palade P, Hsieh JC. Human hairless protein roles in skin/hair and emerging connections to brain and other cancers. J Cell Biochem. 2018;119(1):69–80.
5. Adil A, Godwin M. The effectiveness of treatments for androgenetic alopecia: a systematic review and meta-analysis. J Am Acad Dermatol. 2017;77(1):136–41.

Chapter 22
A Chronic Inflammatory Scalp Disorder with Coexisted Alopecia

Uwe Wollina

A 22-years-old male patient presented with pustules and scarring alopecia (Fig. 22.1) on the scalp since a couple of months. The pustules were painful. Topical corticosteroids were not helpful to control the disease. His medical history was otherwise unremarkable. There was no family history of hair or scalp disorders.

Based on the case description and the photographs, what is your diagnosis?

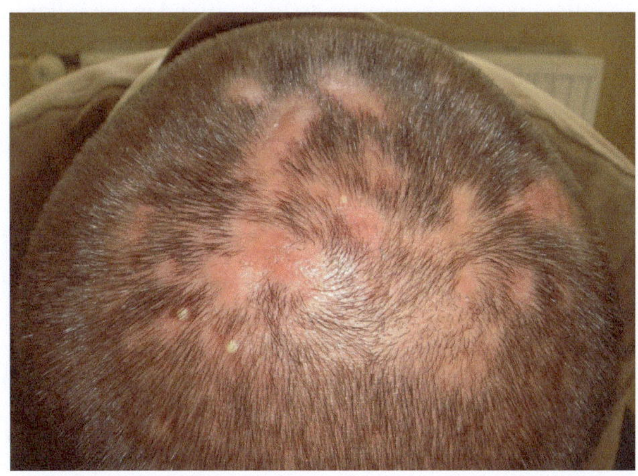

Fig. 22.1 Multiple pustules and alopecic lesions on the scalp

U. Wollina (✉)
Department of Dermatology and Allergology, Städtisches Klinikum Dresden, Academic Teaching Hospital, Dresden, Germany
e-mail: Uwe.Wollina@klinikum-dresden.de

A. Waśkiel-Burnat et al. (eds.), *Clinical Cases in Hair Disorders*, Clinical Cases in Dermatology, https://doi.org/10.1007/978-3-030-93423-1_22

Differential Diagnoses

1. Tinea capitis.
2. Dissecting folliculitis.
3. Folliculitis decalvans.
4. Eosinophilic pustular dermatosis of the scalp.
5. Gram-negative folliculitis.

Diagnosis

Folliculitis decalvans.

Discussion

Folliculitis decalvans is an orphan disease. It is characterized by a chronic and relapsing course of painful follicular papules, pustules, crusting, and tufting of hairs (bundle hairs). The chronic inflammation eventually results in hair follicle destruction, loss of bulge-resident stem cells, and scarring alopecia. Recent studies suggest a persistent unbalanced, subepidermal microbiota with *Staphyloccocus aureus* and an inflammasome activation to be involved in the inflammation and chronicity [1, 2].

The pain is a major symptom to differentiate this disorder from tinea capitis. Gram-negative folliculitis may be painful but often the pain is milder, the inflammation less pronounced. Alopecia is rarely seen with gram-negative folliculitis. Dissecting folliculitis can be coincide with inverse acne (hidradenitis suppurativa) and shows a similar clinical pattern with boils and interconnecting abscesses leading eventually to extensive dermal fibrosis [3].

The treatment of folliculitis decalvans is not standardized. Dapsone and isotretinoin lead to an improvement in up to 60% and 90% respectively. The combination of clindamycin plus rifampicin achieved response rates of about 80% with longer remissions [4]. An early treatment may prevent extensive scarring alopecia. Newer treatment options include biologics such as adalimumab or apremilast [5, 6].

Key Points
- Folliculitis decalvans is a chronic and painful hair disorder of the scalp
- Inflammasome activation and disturbances of the local microbiome are involved in its pathogenesis
- Treatment aims to control inflammation and to prevent scarring alopecia

References

1. Matard B, Donay JL, Resche-Rigon M, Tristan A, Farhi D, Rousseau C, Mercier-Delarue S, Cavelier-Balloy B, Assouly P, Petit A, Bagot M, Reygagne P. Folliculitis decalvans is characterized by a persistent, abnormal subepidermal microbiota. Exp Dermatol. 2020;29(3):295–8.
2. Eyraud A, Milpied B, Thiolat D, Darrigade AS, Boniface K, Taïeb A, Seneschal J. Inflammasome activation characterizes lesional skin of folliculitis decalvans. Acta Derm Venereol. 2018;98(6):570–5.
3. Wolff H, Fischer TW, Blume-Peytavi U. The diagnosis and treatment of hair and scalp diseases. Dtsch Arztebl Int. 2016;113(21):377–86.
4. Rambhia PH, Conic RRZ, Murad A, Atanaskova-Mesinkovska N, Piliang M, Bergfeld W. Updates in therapeutics for folliculitis decalvans: a systematic review with evidence-based analysis. J Am Acad Dermatol. 2019;80(3):794–801.
5. Melo DF, Jorge Machado C, Bordignon NL, da Silva LL, Ramos PM. Lymecycline as a treatment option for dissecting cellulitis and folliculitis decalvans. Dermatol Ther. 2020;33:e14051. https://doi.org/10.1111/dth.14051.
6. Fässler M, Radonjic-Hoesli S, Feldmeyer L, Imstepf V, Pelloni L, Yawalkar N, de Viragh PA. Successful treatment of refractory folliculitis decalvans with apremilast. JAAD Case Rep. 2020;6(10):1079–81.

Chapter 23
An Expanding Patch of Alopecia on the Occipital Scalp in a Male

Sacchelli Lidia, Filippi Federica, Loi Camilla, Pileri Alessandro, and Federico Bardazzi

Clinical History

A 42-year-old, otherwise healthy, Caucasian male came to our observation for consultation regarding an expanding patch of alopecia along the occipital area. The patient complained of moderate pain, especially when lying down in bed during the night. He also reported a wax and wane itch. He was otherwise healthly and denied any trauma or drug assumption before the development of the lesion. In particular, he came to our observation because the patch of alopecia was rapidly expanding from a millimetric round area on the occipital region to a band-like area involving almost the whole back of the neck. Moreover, he reported a reduced quality of life due to the worsening of the pain in the last weeks (Figs. 23.1 and 23.2).

Based upon the history and clinical appearance, what is your diagnosis?

Differential Diagnoses

1. Bacterial folliculitis.
2. Dissecting cellulitis.
3. Folliculitis decalvans.
4. Acne keloidalis nuchae.

S. Lidia · F. Federica · L. Camilla · P. Alessandro (✉) · F. Bardazzi
Dermatology-IRCCS Policlinico di Sant'Orsola, Department of Experimental, Diagnostic and Specialty Medicine (DIMES), Alma Mater Studiorum University of Bologna, Bologna, Italy
e-mail: alessandro.pileri2@unibo.it; federico.bardazzi@aosp.bo.it

© The Author(s), under exclusive license to Springer Nature Switzerland AG 2022
A. Waśkiel-Burnat et al. (eds.), *Clinical Cases in Hair Disorders*, Clinical Cases in Dermatology, https://doi.org/10.1007/978-3-030-93423-1_23

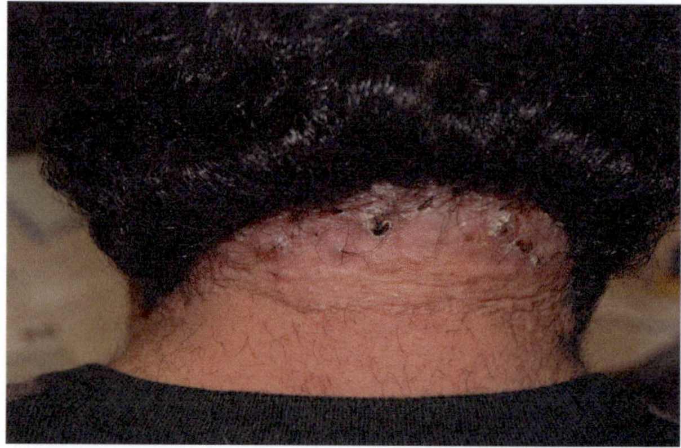

Fig. 23.1 A band-like patch of alopecia along the occipital region of the scalp

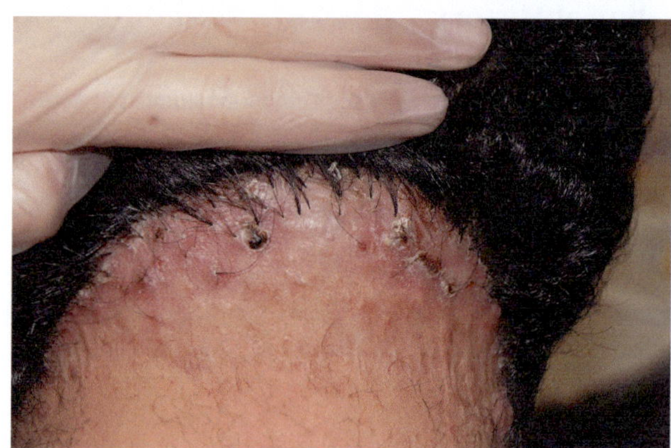

Fig. 23.2 Close-up view of the scarring alopecia area of the back of the neck. Diffuse follicular pustules and tufted hair on an erythematous background are present

Diagnosis

Folliculitis decalvans.

Discussion

Folliculitis decalvans (FD) is the most common type of neutrophilic scarring alopecia. It is typically associated with symptoms such as pain and itch, along with signs like purulent discharge and erythematous patches [1]. FD may involve any area of the scalp with a multifocal distribution [1]. However, the beard, face or limbs could also be involved, alone or in association with FD of the scalp [2]. The etiology is still unknown but several theories consider the role of *Staphylococcus aureus*, whose superantigens may cause activation of T lymphocytes, and the release of inflammatory cytokines resulting in follicular destruction [3]. Moreover, a defect of the epidermal barrier seems to contribute to FD chronicity along with an impaired phagocytosis [4]. Genetic predisposition might be present, as some familial cases have been described [1].

FD is a primary scarring alopecia since the inflammatory process targets the hair follicle itself, resulting in permanent hair loss [1]. Most cases involve adult males, with a male to female ratio varying from 1.3:1 to 6.5:1 [5]. However, both sexes may develop FD, as well as children [5].

Clinical features depend on the activity of the disease. Active lesions are represented by areas of scarring alopecia with multiple pustules at the periphery; the surface of these areas is smooth and follicular orifices are absent. Moreover, some tufted hair might be detected at the periphery of the patch of alopecia as in our patient [6]. Sometimes, a variable amount of scale could be visible [7]. By contrast, chronic lesions lack pustules could be associated with an erythematous background or scale [6].

On trichoscopy, FD shows cicatricial whitish patches without follicular ostia, perifollicular erythema and scale, anisotrichosis and follicular pustules that could be used for diagnosis and for monitoring the disease activity [8].

Sometimes a deep, subcutaneous biopsy might be necessary to rule out the forms of cicatricial alopecia-like lymphocytic cicatricial alopecia, such as lichen planus pilaris, discoid lupus erythematosus and central centrifugal cicatricial alopecia [9]. Active lesions show neutrophilic follicular pustules and foreign body giant cells in the superficial and mid dermis, while chronic specimens present few neutrophils and more plasma-cells along with abundant fibrosis [9].

Differential diagnosis for FD includes: dissecting cellulitis of the scalp, acne keloidalis nuchae, erosive pustular dermatosis of the scalp and kerion [6, 7].

Antibiotics are the therapeutic gold standard [10]. Bacterial cultures of pustules testing antibiotics sensitivity should be performed in all patients [10]. Cycles of tetracyclines have been proposed along with high-potency topical corticosteroids, as in our patient, who was treated with doxycycline 100 mg twice a day and clobetasol propionate 0.05% once a day for 10 weeks. Moreover, as in our case, most patients experience a recurrence of the FD after drug discontinuation. In this case, it is wise to restart therapy until control is achieved once again [10]. In recalcitrant cases, rifampicin and or clindamycin might be considered as well as oral isotretinoin, systemic corticosteroids, dapsone or TNF-a inhibitors [11, 12].

Key Points
- Folliculitis decalvans is the most common type of neutrophilic scarring alopecia which is typically associated with symptoms such as pain and itch along with signs like purulent discharge and erythematous patches
- It typically occurs in men and involves the scalp
- Diagnosis could be clinical but sometimes biopsy might be helpful to differentiate FD from other forms of cicatrial alopecial, especially lymphocytic types
- Therapy consists of antibiotics, but might be challenging to achieve a durable remission of the disease as it frequently recurs at drug suspension

References

1. Otberg N, Kang H, Alzolibani AA, Shapiro J. Folliculitis decalvans. Dermatol Ther. 2008;21:238–44.
2. Yang A, Hannaford R, Kossard S. Folliculitis decalvans-like pustular plaques on the limbs sparing the scalp. Australas J Dermatol. 2020;61:54–6.
3. Matard B, Donay JL, Resche-Rigon M, Tristan A, Farhi D, Rousseau C, Mercier-Delarue S, Cavelier-Balloy B, Assouly P, Petit A, Bagot M, Reygagne P. Folliculitis decalvans is characterized by a persistent, abnormal subepidermal microbiota. Exp Dermatol. 2020;29:295–8.
4. Whiting DA. Cicatricial alopecia: clinico-pathological findings and treatment. Clin Dermatol. 2001;19:211–25.
5. Chandrawansa PH, Giam YC. Folliculitis decalvans: a retrospective study in a tertiary referred centre, over five years. Singap Med J. 2003;44:84–7.
6. Tan E, Martinka M, Ball N, Shapiro J. Primary cicatricial alopecias: clinicopathology of 112 cases. J Am Acad Dermatol. 2004;50:25–32.
7. Powell J, Dawber RP. Folliculitis decalvans and tufted folliculitis are specific infective diseases that may lead to scarring, but are not a subset of central centrifugal scarring alopecia. Arch Dermatol. 2001;137:373–4.
8. Saceda-Corralo D, Moreno-Arrones OM, Rodrigues-Barata R, Rubio-Lombraña M, Mir-Bonafé JF, Morales-Raya C, Miguel-Gómez L, Hermosa-Gelbard Á, Jaén-Olasolo P, Vañó-Galván S. Trichoscopy activity scale for folliculitis decalvans. J Eur Acad Dermatol Venereol. 2020;34:e55–7.
9. Stefanato CM. Histopathology of alopecia: a clinicopathological approach to diagnosis. Histopathology. 2010;56:24–38.
10. Miguel-Gómez L, Rodrigues-Barata AR, Molina-Ruiz A, Martorell-Calatayud A, Fernández-Crehuet P, Grimalt R, Barco D, Arias-Santiago S, Serrano-Falcón C, Camacho FM, Saceda-Corralo D, Jaén-Olasolo P, Vañó-Galván S. Folliculitis decalvans: effectiveness of therapies and prognostic factors in a multicenter series of 60 patients with long-term follow-up. J Am Acad Dermatol. 2018;79:878–83.
11. Paquet P, Piérard GE. Traitement par dapsone de la folliculite décalvante [Dapsone treatment of folliculitis decalvans]. Ann Dermatol Venereol. 2004;131:195–7.
12. Kreutzer K, Effendy I. Therapy-resistant folliculitis decalvans and lichen planopilaris successfully treated with adalimumab. J Dtsch Dermatol Ges. 2014;12:74–6.

Chapter 24
An Extensive Alopecia Associated with Scaly Plaques of the Scalp

Diego Abbenante, Federico Bardazzi, Camilla Loi, Miriam Anna Carpanese, and Michelangelo La Placa

A 32-year-old woman with severe scalp dermatitis and alopecia was referred to our Unit from the Department of Gastroenterology. Her personal and family history was negative for skin or rheumatic disorders.

The patient's medical record was relevant for ulcerative colitis (UC) diagnosed eight years before, for which she had been previously treated with mesalazine and systemic steroid courses. Due to poor control of the disease, the gastroenterologists decided to start therapy with an induction dose of adalimumab 160 mg at week 0 followed by 80 mg after two weeks and then 40 mg every two weeks. Cutaneous lesions appeared about three months after the first administration of the biological drug.

Based upon the history and clinical appearance, what is your diagnosis?

Differential Diagnoses

1. Seborrheic dermatitis.
2. Paradoxical scalp psoriasis with alopecia.
3. Mycosis fungoides.
4. Tinea capitis.

Diagnosis: Paradoxical scalp psoriasis with alopecia.

A physical examination revealed thick hyperkeratotic plaques covering the entire scalp surface with severe alopecia (Fig. 24.1). Other well-defined, erythematous,

D. Abbenante · F. Bardazzi (✉) · C. Loi · M. A. Carpanese · M. La Placa
Dermatology Unit, IRCCS Azienda Ospedaliero-Universitaria di Bologna, Bologna, Italy
e-mail: diego.abbenante@studio.unibo.it; federico.bardazzi@aosp.bo.it; michelangelo.laplaca@unibo.it

A. Waśkiel-Burnat et al. (eds.), *Clinical Cases in Hair Disorders*, Clinical Cases in Dermatology, https://doi.org/10.1007/978-3-030-93423-1_24

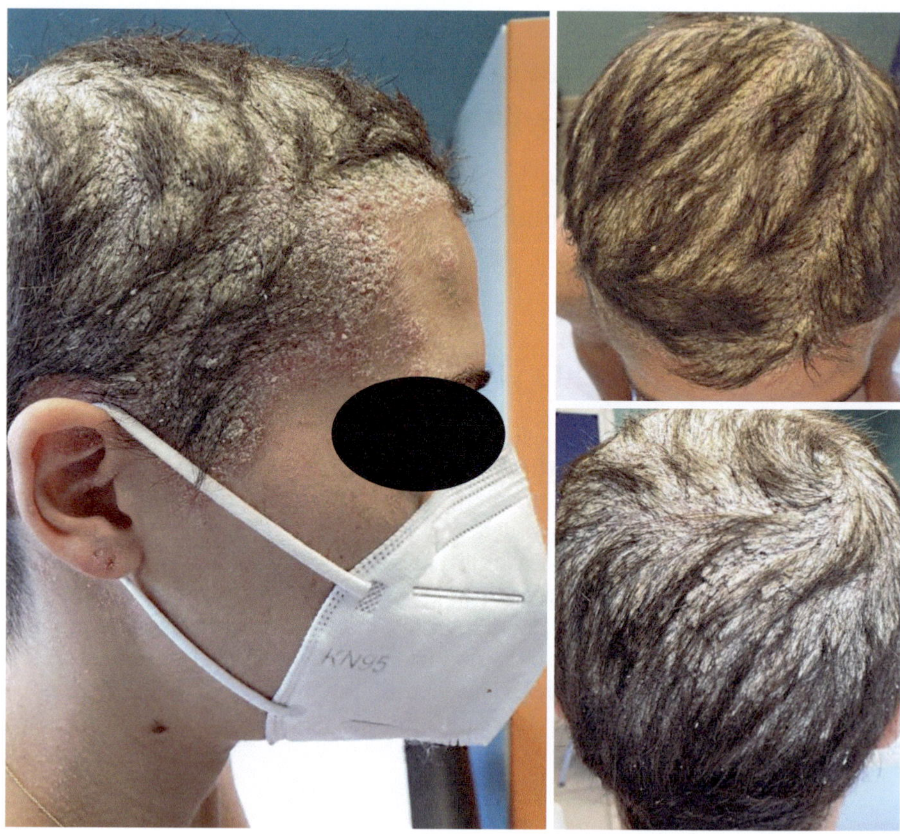

Fig. 24.1 An extensive alopecia associated with scaly plaques of the scalp

scaly plaques were diffused on the trunk and palmoplantar regions. A gentle scrape of one lesion revealed punctate bleeding points (positive Auspitz sign). Mild, bilateral, symmetric, cervical adenopathy was present. Routine blood tests were within the normal ranges except for C-reactive protein (CRP) 4.2 mg/L (n.v. <3.0 mg/L).

Based on the patient's history and clinical findings, a diagnosis of Paradoxical Psoriasis (PP) induced by anti-TNFα treatment was made.

In the first instance, topical therapies were started. The patient applied 10% salicylic acid ointment under cellophane occlusion overnight. In the morning, after washing her hair with clobetasol propionate 0.05% shampoo, she applied betamethasone dipropionate/calcipotriol lotion on all lesions. Treatment with adalimumab was discontinued, and ustekinumab was initiated to treat UC. Both the alopecia and scalp psoriasis significantly improved after five weeks of therapy, so topical products were progressively tapered and then discontinued. The patient's inflammatory bowel disease remains well controlled and there has been no resurgence of either alopecia or psoriasis.

Discussion

Anti-TNFα drugs have been shown to be effective for maintaining stable remission in patients with inflammatory bowel diseases and are widely used in the treatment of psoriasis as well as in many inflammatory conditions. PP is defined as a peculiar type of psoriasis that may occur de novo or as the exacerbation of pre-existent psoriasis during treatment with biological drugs or in patients with relatives affected by psoriasis [1].

The first case of PP induced by anti-TNFα was described in 2004 [2]. The prevalence of PP in patients treated with anti-TNFα is around 2–5%, with a predilection for women. The most frequent clinical presentation is plaque psoriasis or palmoplantar pustular psoriasis, while severe scalp involvement with alopecia is seen in 7.5% of cases [3].

The exact mechanism of TNFα inhibitor-induced psoriasis remains elusive, however some studies have hypothesized that, in subjects with genetic predisposition, TNF blockade may allow unexpected IFN-α production by plasmacytoid dendritic cells which would cause the migration of T cells to the skin, resulting in a psoriasiform reaction [4].

Concerning the treatment of paradoxical psoriasis, a recent study highlights that remission was achieved in 64% of patients with topical treatment alone, with no need for any additional treatment or discontinuation of the anti-TNFα drugs. For patients who failed to respond to topical agents, ustekinumab (a human monoclonal antibody directed against IL-12 and IL-23) showed efficacy in all subjects, achieving a good control of both the inflammatory bowel disease and the cutaneous condition [5].

Patients with PP may develop a non-scarring alopecia as a result of scalp involvement. However, if not properly treated, psoriasiform alopecia can lead to permanent hair loss [6, 7]. Despite the fact that this condition has rarely been reported in the medical literature, it is very important to recognize anti-TNF-α-induced scalp psoriasis in order to provide the patient with timely and appropriate treatment.

Key Points
- Paradoxical psoriasis may occur de novo or as the exacerbation of pre-existent psoriasis during treatment with biological drugs
- If not promptly treated, scalp psoriasis can lead to a scarring alopecia
- The classical topical therapy of psoriasis is usually effective in this condition
- In case of topical treatment failure, ustekinumab is effective for both the inflammatory bowel disease and the cutaneous condition

References

1. Bucalo A, Rega F, Zangrilli A, et al. Paradoxical psoriasis induced by anti-TNFα treatment: evaluation of disease-specific clinical and genetic markers. Int J Mol Sci. 2020;21(21):7873.
2. Dereure O, Guillot B, Jorgensen C, Cohen JD, Combes B, Guilhou JJ. Psoriatic lesions induced by antitumour necrosis factor-alpha treatment: two cases. Br J Dermatol. 2004;151(2):506–7.
3. Brown G, Wang E, Leon A, et al. Tumor necrosis factor-α inhibitor-induced psoriasis: systematic review of clinical features, histopathological findings, and management experience. J Am Acad Dermatol. 2017;76(2):334–41.
4. Iborra M, Beltrán B, Bastida G, Aguas M, Nos P. Infliximab and adalimumab-induced psoriasis in Crohn's disease: a paradoxical side effect. J Crohns Colitis. 2011;5(2):157–61.
5. Koumaki D, Koumaki V, Katoulis A, et al. Adalimumab-induced scalp psoriasis with severe alopecia as a paradoxical effect in a patient with Crohn's disease successfully treated with ustekinumab. Dermatol Ther. 2020;33(4):e13791.
6. El Shabrawi-Caelen L, La Placa M, Vincenzi C, Haidn T, Muellegger R, Tosti A. Adalimumab-induced psoriasis of the scalp with diffuse alopecia: a severe potentially irreversible cutaneous side effect of TNF-alpha blockers. Inflamm Bowel Dis. 2010;16(2):182–3.
7. Bardazzi F, Fanti PA, Orlandi C, Chieregato C, Misciali C. Psoriatic scarring alopecia: observations in four patients. Int J Dermatol. 1999;38(10):765–8.

Chapter 25
A 58-Year-Old Man with Alopecia on the Frontal Area

Amr M. Ammar, Shady M. Ibrahim, and Mohamed L. Elsaie

A 58-year-old man presented with hair loss on the frontal area of the scalp.

A physical examination revealed recession of the frontotemporal and occipital hair line. Moreover, eyebrow loss was presented (Fig. 25.1).

Dermoscopy showed loss of follicular openings and transparent proximal hair shaft emergence, which are segments of the proximal hair shafts that are visible underneath the skin. Moreover, patches of pale atrophic skin with the absence of vellus hairs and perifollicular pustules were observed. Very fine, less adherent hair casts, multiple irregular white dots in addition to regular white dots were also detected (Figs. 25.2, 25.3, and 25.4).

Based on the case description and the photographs, what is your diagnosis?

Differential Diagnoses

1. Alopecia areata (ophiasis pattern).
2. Frontal fibrosing alopecia.
3. Discoid lupus erythematosus.
4. Dissecting cellulitis of the scalp.

A. M. Ammar · S. M. Ibrahim
Department of Dermatology and Venerology, Al-Azhar University, Cairo, Egypt

M. L. Elsaie (✉)
Department of Dermatology and Venereology, National Research Center, Cairo, Egypt

A. Waśkiel-Burnat et al. (eds.), *Clinical Cases in Hair Disorders*, Clinical Cases in Dermatology, https://doi.org/10.1007/978-3-030-93423-1_25

Fig. 25.1 A 58-year-old man with recession of the frontotemporal hair line

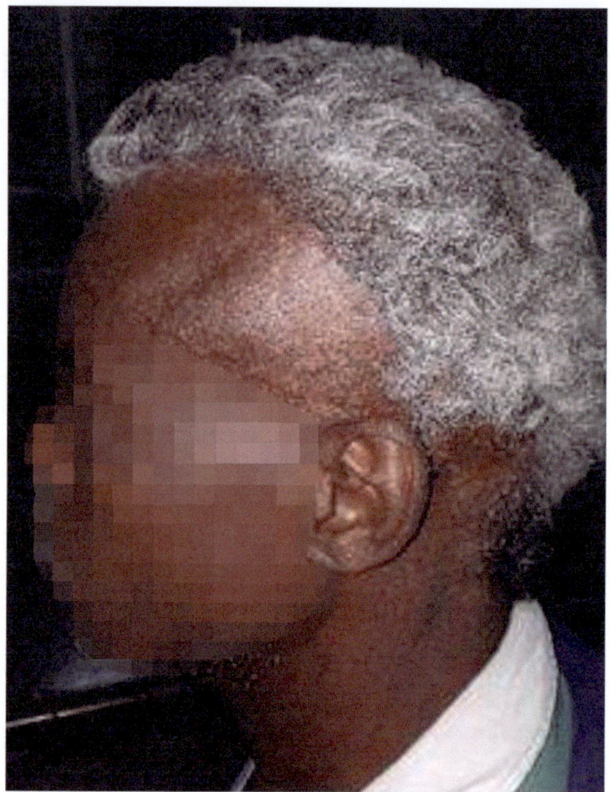

Fig. 25.2 Dermoscopy shows loss of follicular openings, perifollicular scaling, the absence of vellus hairs. There are very fine, less adherent hair casts around hair shafts and multiple irregular white dots

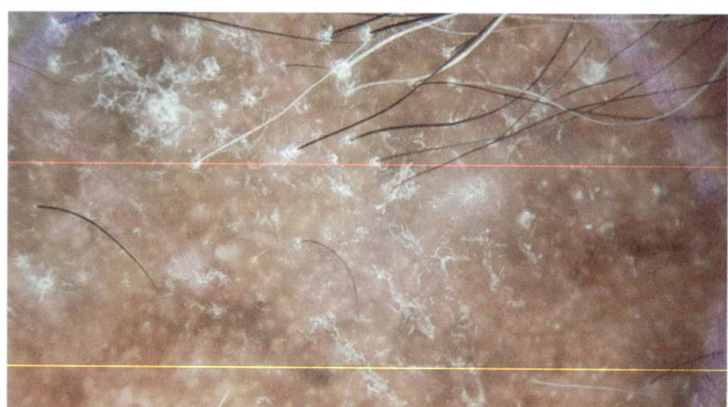

Fig. 25.3 Dermoscopy with the presence of multiple irregular white dots, and regular white dots

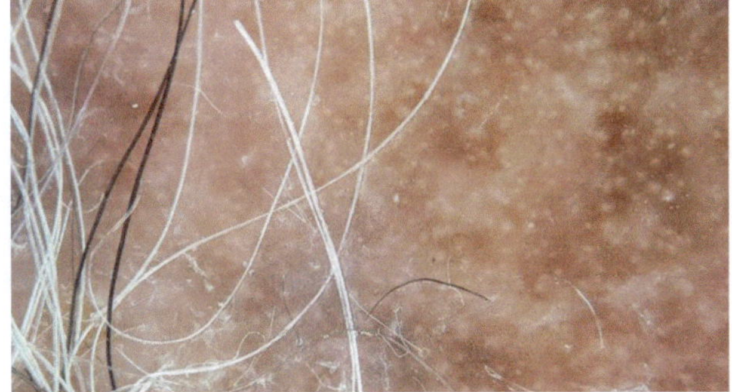

Fig. 25.4 Dermoscopy shows large perifollicular pustule without tufting

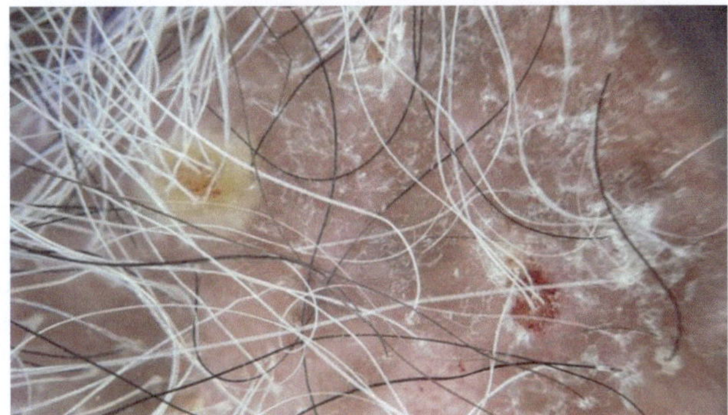

Diagnosis

Frontal fibrosing alopecia.

Discussion

Frontal fibrosing alopecia (FFA) is a form of cicatricial alopecia. By the time the patient seeks medical advice part of the hair/eyebrows are usually permanently lost. This disease is, in fact, difficult to recognize in its debut because it is subtle and usually slowly progressive and patients often attribute their hair/eyebrow loss to aging, delaying medical consultation. Early recognition of the disorder would allow early treatment and eventually prevent disease progression.

FFA is much more common in postmenopausal females, but cases in young women and, more rarely, in men have been reported [1, 2].

FFA has been reported more frequently in Caucasian patients, but over the years several cases of African American [3, 4] and Asian [5] patients have also been described, probably previously misdiagnosed as traction alopecia, androgenetic alopecia, or alopecia areata.

FFA is a cicatricial alopecia and this means that the hair follicles are permanently replaced by a scar-like fibrous tissue. In FFA, as in classic lichen planopilaris (LPP), the infundibulo-isthmic (bulge) region of the hair follicle is attacked by an immune-mediated inflammatory infiltrate, characterized by a prevalence of CD8+ T lymphocytes [6, 7].

Inflammation of the bulge area destroys the hair follicle stem cells, preventing hair regeneration. It has been hypothesized that loss of the follicular immune privilege, as in alopecia areata, and a peroxisome proliferatoractivated receptor (PPAR)-γ deficiency might enable the inflammatory process to attack the stem cells in the bulge region and permanently destroy them [8].

Three clinical patterns of hair loss in FFA have been described, according to the different types of hairline recession described over the years [9]: linear, diffuse zig-zag, and pseudo-fringe. The linear pattern is the band of uniform frontal hairline recession in the absence of loss of hair density behind the hairline. The diffuse zig-zag pattern is the same as linear but with at least 50% decreased hair density. Pseudo-fringe hairline recession is a clinical presentation similar to traction alopecia (hence the term 'pseudo') where the fringe sign is the presence of some hair retained along the hairline (especially on the temporal area) ahead of the alopecic skin [10].

Trichoscopy (scalp dermoscopy) is a valid aid in doubtful cases/limited disease or when the eyebrows are the sole localization of the disease [11]. Even a handheld dermoscope reveals the cicatricial nature of this alopecia, showing reduced/absent follicular openings. Follicular hyperkeratosis (peripilar casts) and perifollicular erythema are seen around terminal hairs, but they may be very subtle. These are signs of active inflammation, but not necessarily signs of disease progression [12, 13]. The absence of vellus hair is diagnostic and allows fast differentiation of FFA from androgenetic alopecia.

Treatment may differ according to the disease localization, disease stage, and presence of inflammation and itch. Treatment may also change over time, depending on the patient's response. Many studies demonstrated follicular inflammation around the infundibulum-isthmic region of the clinically unaffected scalp of FFA patients, indicating that treatment should involve the whole scalp [14].

Key Points
- Frontal fibrosing alopecia is a cicatricial alopecia and by the time the patient seeks medical advice part of the hair/eyebrows are usually permanently lost
- Inflammation of the bulge area destroys the hair follicle stem cells, preventing hair regeneration

References

1. Vano-Galvan S, Molina-Riuz AM, Serrano-Falcon C, et al. Frontal fibrosing alopecia: a multi-center review of 355 patients. J Am Acad Dermatol. 2014;70:670–8.

2. Alegre-Sánchez A, Saceda-Corralo D, Bernárdez C, et al. Frontal fibrosing alopecia in male patients: a report of 12 cases. J Eur Acad Dermatol Venereol. 2017;31:e112–4.
3. Miteva M, Whiting D, Harries M, et al. Frontal fibrosing alopecia in black patients. Br J Dermatol. 2012;167:208–10.
4. Dlova N, Jordaan HF, Skenjane A, et al. Frontal fibrosing alopecia: a clinical review of 20 black patients from South Africa. Br J Dermatol. 2013;169:939–41.
5. Inui S, Nakajima T, Shono F, Itami S. Dermoscopic findings in frontal fibrosing alopecia: report of four cases. Int J Dermatol. 2008;47:796–9.
6. Kossard S, Lee MS, Wilkinson B. Postmenopausal frontalfibrosing alopecia: a frontal variant of lichen planopilaris. J Am Acad Dermatol. 1997;36:59–66.
7. Ma SA, Imadojemu S, Beer K, et al. Inflammatory features of frontal fibrosing alopecia. J Cutan Pathol. 2017;44:672–6.
8. Karnik P, Tekeste Z, McCormick TS, et al. Hair follicle stem cell-specific PPAR-γ deletion causes scarring alopecia. J Investig Dermatol. 2009;129:1243–57.
9. Moreno-Arrones OM, Saceda-Corralo D, Fonda-Pascual P, et al. Frontal fibrosing alopecia: clinical and prognostic classification. J Eur Acad Dermatol Venereol. 2017;31:1739–45.
10. Pirmez R, Duque-Estrada B, Abraham LS, et al. It's not all traction: the pseudo 'fringe sign' in frontal fibrosing alopecia. Br J Dermatol. 2015;173:1336–8.
11. Waśkiel-Burnat A, Rakowska A, Kurzeja M, et al. The value of dermoscopy in diagnosing eyebrow loss in patients with alopecia areata and frontal fibrosing alopecia. J Eur Acad Dermatol Venereol. 2018;33(1):213–9. https://doi.org/10.1111/jdv.15279.
12. Toledo-Pastrana T, Garcia-Hernandez MJ, Camacho-Martinez F. Perifollicular erythema as trichoscopy sign of progression in frontal fibrosing alopecia. Int J Trichol. 2013;5:151–3.
13. Fernandez-Crehuet P, Rodrigues-Barata AR, Vano-Galvan S, et al. Trichoscopic features of frontal fibrosing alopecia: results in 249 patients. J Am Acad Dermatol. 2015;72:357–9.
14. Doche I, Valente NS, Romiti R, Hordinsky M. "Normal-appearing" scalp areas are also affected in lichen planopilaris and frontal fibrosing alopecia: an observational histopathologic study of 40 patients. Clin Exp Dermatol. 2018;29(3):278–81. https://doi.org/10.1111/exd.13834.

Chapter 26
A 68-Year-Old Woman with Frontal Scarring Alopecia

Özge Aşkın, Server Serdaroğlu, and Zekayi Kutlubay

A 68-year-old female presented to the dermatology with one year history of hair loss especially on the frontal area of the scalp. She also reported thinning and shedding on her both eyebrows.

A physical examination revealed frontal and temporal recession of the hairlines with perifollicular erythema. Bilateral thinning of eyebrows and partial alopecia on the left eyebrow were also observed (Figs. 26.1, 26.2, and 26.3).

In histopathological examination, loss of hair follicles, perifollicular fibrosis and mild lymphocytic infiltration around hair follicles were seen (Figs. 26.4 and 26.5a, b).

Based on the case description and the photograph, what is your diagnosis?

Differential Diagnoses

1. Discoid lupus erythematosus.
2. Female pattern hair loss.
3. Frontal fibrosing alopecia.
4. Alopecia areata.
5. Traction alopecia.

Ö. Aşkın · S. Serdaroğlu · Z. Kutlubay (✉)
Cerrahpaşa Medical Faculty, Department of Dermatology, Istanbul University-Cerrahpaşa, Istanbul, Turkey

© The Author(s), under exclusive license to Springer Nature Switzerland AG 2022
A. Waśkiel-Burnat et al. (eds.), *Clinical Cases in Hair Disorders*, Clinical Cases in Dermatology, https://doi.org/10.1007/978-3-030-93423-1_26

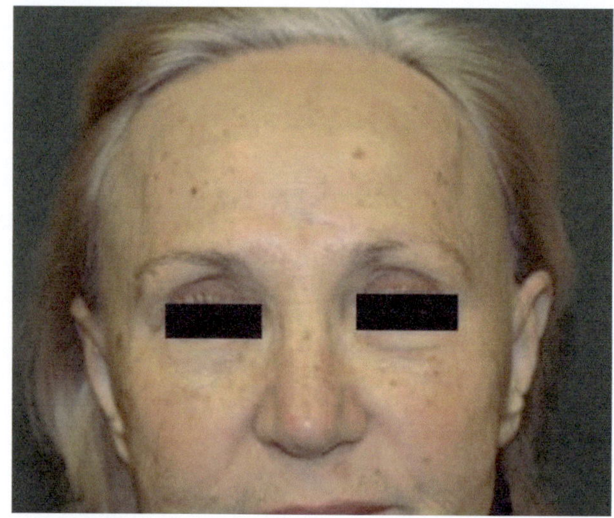

Fig. 26.1 Frontal recession of the hairline. Bilateral thinning of eyebrows and partial alopecia on the left eyebrow are observed

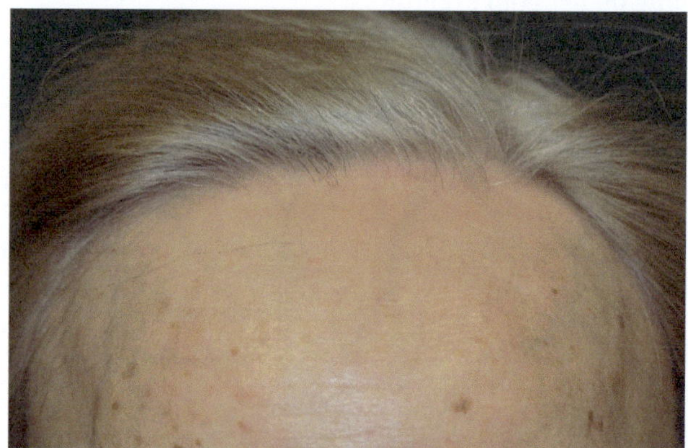

Fig. 26.2 Frontal recession of the hairlines with perifollicular erythema. There is "lonely hair sign" on the frontal area

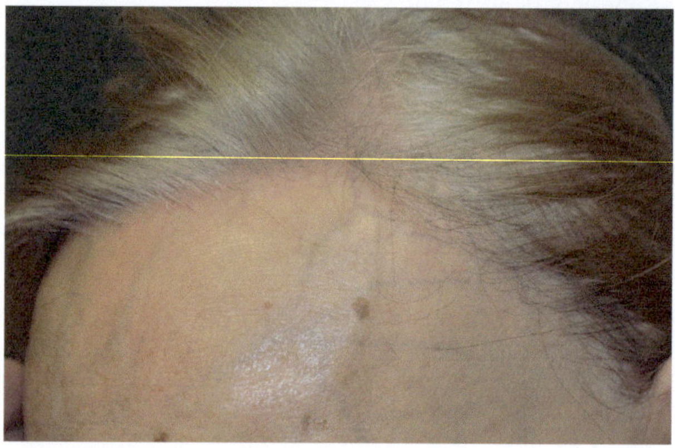

Fig. 26.3 Temporal recession of hair line and hair loss and thinning on the temporal area

Fig. 26.4 Histology shows loss of hair follicles, fibrosis and mild lymphocytic infiltration around one hair follicle (×200, H&E)

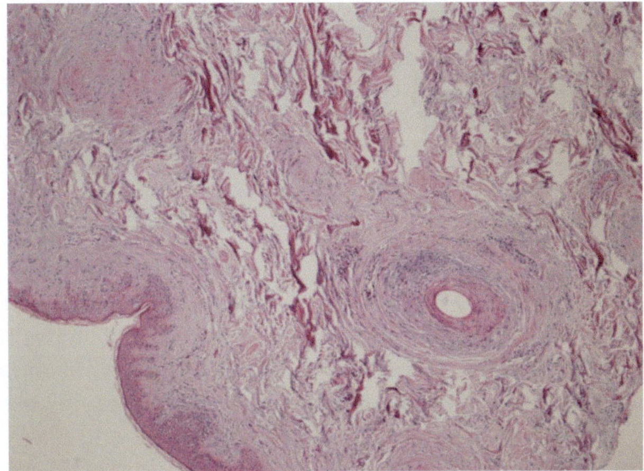

Fig. 26.5 (**a**, **b**) Histology shows mild lymphocytic infiltration around hair follicles and perfollicular fibrosis (×400, H&E)

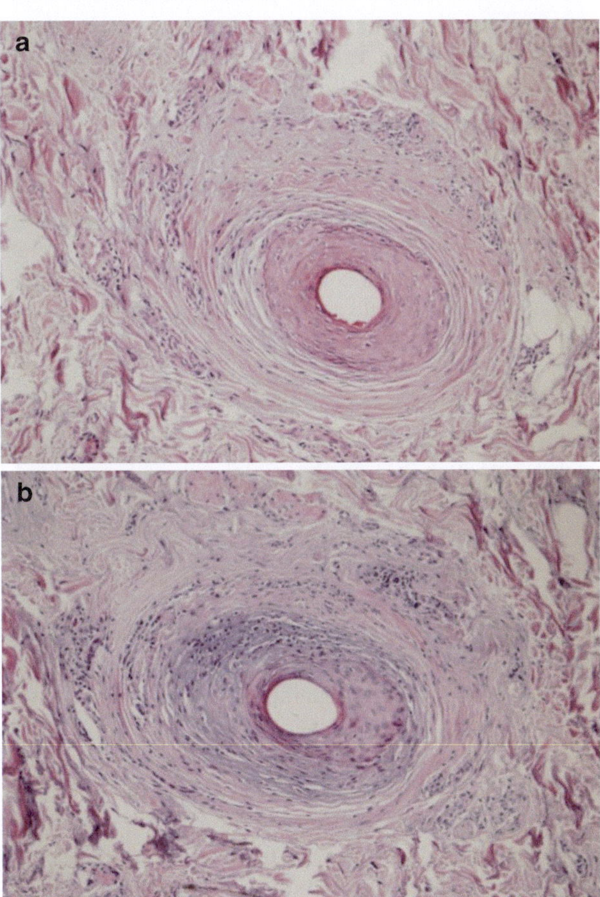

Diagnosis

Frontal fibrosing alopecia.

Discussion

Frontal fibrosing alopecia (FFA) is a form of primary lymphocytic cicatricial alopecia characterized by progressive involvement of the frontotemporal hairline and eyebrows. It is considered as a variant of lichen planopilaris on the basis of its clinical and histological features. FFA is seen mostly in postmenopausal females [1, 2].

Hormonal effects, genetic predisposition, and environmental factors have been thought to play a role in the etiopathogenesis of FFA [3]. The clinical features of FFA are very distinctive. FFA presents mainly as a band-like recession of the frontotemporal hairline with lighter skin compared to the forehead and the absence of follicular ostia. Within the frontotemporal hairline, perifollicular erythema and fine scale are present [1, 3]. On dermatoscopic evaluation, big irregular white dots, peripilar white scales, peripilar erythema and lack of follicular ostia may be seen. FFA has a chronic course. Stabilization of the disease may occur spontaneously or be induced by treatment. Eyelash loss, facial papules, and body hair involvement indicate severe form of FFA while eyebrow involvement is associated with milder FFA [4].

Histopathologic features of FFA are similar to lichen pilanopilaris and show different presentations according to the stage at diagnosis. Perifollicular fibrosis and lymphohistiocytic infiltrate around the infundibulum and isthmus region are seen. The late stage is characterized by more severe perifollicular fibrosis, with reduced follicular density until scar tissue replaces the pilosebaceous units [1, 4].

In differential diagnosis of FFA, alopecia areata, androgenetic alopecia, lupus erythematosus and tractional alopecia should be considered. The sudden onset of progressive hair loss on the scalp and eyebrows lead to alopecia areata. In lupus erythematosus, hyperkeratinization with mottled hyperpigmentation and hypopigmentation are seen. Androgenetic alopecia in women usually spares the frontal hairline. Traction alopecia causes also hair loss localized to the frontal hairline with broken hairs of uneven lengths [5].

Common initial therapies for FFA include local therapies (topical corticosteroids, topical calcineurin inhibitors, intralesional corticosteroid injections, topical minoxidil) and systemic therapies (oral 5-alpha reductase inhibitors, hydroxychloroquine, systemic corticosteroids and oral tetracyclines). Combination therapy is more beneficial than monotherapy. Intralesional corticosteroids and 5a-reductase inhibitors (finasteride and dutasteride) are the most efficacious options for the treatment of FFA [6, 7].

The presented patient was diagnosed with FFA. We started high-potency topical corticosteroid, topical minoxidil and finasteride 2.5 mg daily.

Key Points
1. Frontal fibrosing alopecia is a form of primary lymphocytic cicatricial alopecia that is a variant of lichen planopilaris
2. Frontotemporal region of the scalp and the eyebrows are mostly effected
3. The course of frontal fibrosing alopecia is usually slow and stable
4. Intralesional corticosteroids and 5a-reductase inhibitors might be effective at preventing the progression of hair loss

References

1. Iorizzo M, Tosti A. Frontal Fibrosing alopecia: an update on pathogenesis, diagnosis, and treatment. Am J Clin Dermatol. 2019;20(3):379–90. https://doi.org/10.1007/s40257-019-00424-y.
2. Moreno-Arrones OM, Saceda-Corralo D, Fonda-Pascual P, Rodrigues-Barata AR, Buendía-Castaño D, et al. Frontal fibrosing alopecia: clinical and prognostic classification. J Eur Acad Dermatol Venereol. 2017;31(10):1739–45. https://doi.org/10.1111/jdv.14287.
3. To D, Beecker J. Frontal Fibrosing alopecia: update and review of challenges and successes. J Cutan Med Surg. 2018;22(2):182–9. https://doi.org/10.1177/1203475417736279.
4. Bolduc C, Sperling LC, Shapiro J. Primary cicatricial alopecia: lymphocytic primary cicatricial alopecias, including chronic cutaneous lupus erythematosus, lichen planopilaris, frontal fibrosing alopecia, and Graham-Little syndrome. J Am Acad Dermatol. 2016;75(6):1081–99. https://doi.org/10.1016/j.jaad.2014.09.058.
5. Kossard S, Lee MS, Wilkinson B. Postmenopausal frontal fibrosing alopecia: a frontal variant of lichen planopilaris. J Am Acad Dermatol. 1997;36(1):59–66.
6. Gamret AC, Potluri VS, Krishnamurthy K, Fertig RM. Frontal fibrosing alopecia: efficacy of treatment modalities. Int J Women's Health. 2019;29(11):273–85. https://doi.org/10.2147/IJWH.S177308.
7. Ho A, Shapiro J. Medical therapy for frontal fibrosing alopecia: a review and clinical approach. J Am Acad Dermatol. 2019;81(2):568–80. https://doi.org/10.1016/j.jaad.2019.03.079.

Chapter 27
The scalp Infection and with Scarring Alopecia

Tutty Ariani, Satya Wydya Yenny, Yosse Rizal, and Indah Kencana

A seven-year-old boy was referred to the Department of Dermatology and Venereology because pus-filled nodules covered by blackish brown crusts with coexisted scarring alopecia (Fig. 27.1). He also complained of pain, mild fever and hair loss.

Based on the case description and the photographs, what is your diagnosis?

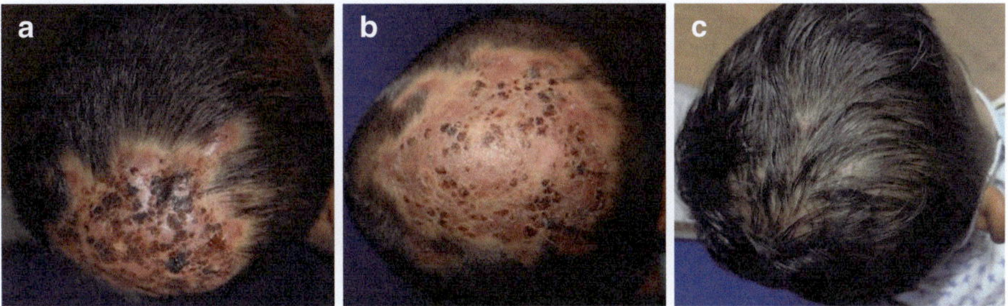

Fig. 27.1 A seven-year boy with the scalp infection and scarring alopecia. (**a**) Blackish brown crusts and multiple erythematous nodules, (**b**) after four weeks of treatment, (**c**) after eight weeks of treatment

T. Ariani · S. W. Yenny (✉) · Y. Rizal · I. Kencana
Department of Dermatology and Venereology, Faculty of Medicine, Universitas Andalas, Padang, Indonesia

Dr. M. Djamil Hospital, Padang, Indonesia

Indonesian Society of Dermatology and Venereology, Jakarta, Indonesia
e-mail: satyawidyayenny@med.unand.ac.id

© The Author(s), under exclusive license to Springer Nature Switzerland AG 2022
A. Waśkiel-Burnat et al. (eds.), *Clinical Cases in Hair Disorders*, Clinical Cases in Dermatology, https://doi.org/10.1007/978-3-030-93423-1_27

Differential Diagnoses

1. Tinea capitis kerion type.
2. Folliculitis decalvans.
3. Seborrheic dermatitis.
4. Dissecting cellulitis.

Diagnosis

Tinea capitis kerion type.

On dermoscopy, blackish brown crusts, comma hairs and bar code-like hairs hairs were presented (Fig. 27.2). A Wood's lamp examination showed green fluorescence (Fig. 27.3a). A potassium hydroxide examination of the scalp lesion showed hyphae and arthrospores (Fig. 27.3b). In fungal culture, *Microsporum canis* was isolated (Fig. 27.3c).

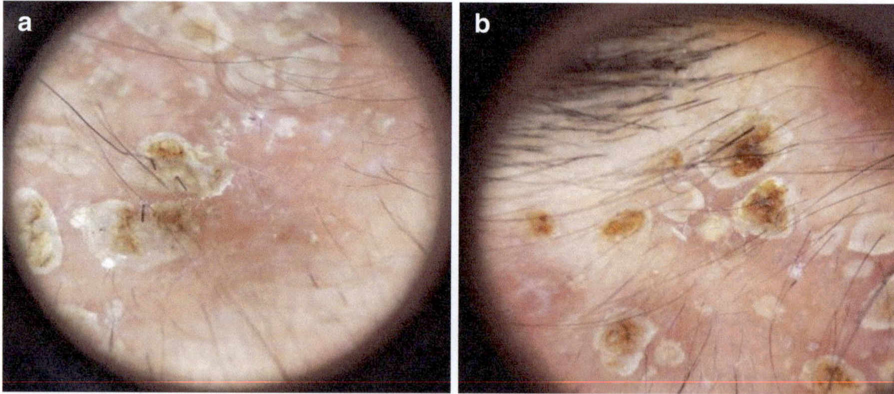

Fig. 27.2 A dermoscopic examination. (**a**) Dermoscopy before treatment shows blackish brown crusts, comma hairs and bar code-like hairs hairs. (**b**) Dermoscopy four weeks after the treatment initation shows a decreased number of blackish brown crusts and numerous vellus hairs

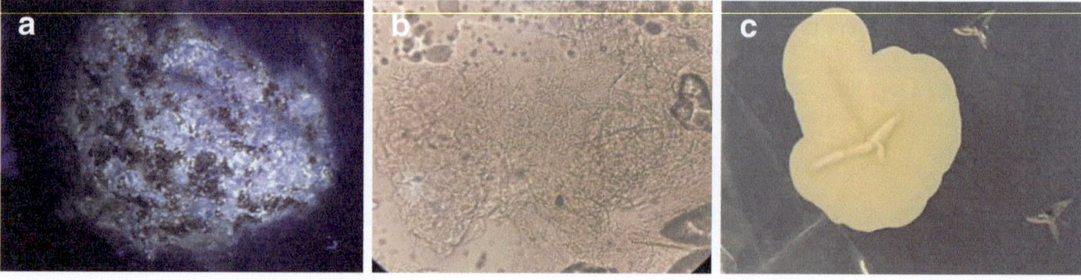

Fig. 27.3 (**a**) A Wood's lamp examination with green fluorescence. (**b**) A potassium hydroxide examination shows hyphae and arthrospora. (**c**) A fungal culture shows *Microsporum canis*

Based on the clinical presentation, dermoscopy and mycological finding, the presented patient was diagnosed with Tinea Capitis Kerion Type.

We started the treatment with griseovulfin 500 mg a day for six–eight weeks (minimally) until three–four months depends on clinical and mycology finding, prednisone 15 mg a day and erythromycin 3 × 200 mg a day for short course, cetirizine syrup 5 mg a day, and ketoconazole 2% cream twice a day with good improvement. A dermoscopic examination four weeks after the treatment initiation showed vellus hair.

Discussion

Kerion represents the inflammatory form of tinea capitis (TC) caused by the hypersensitivity reaction to the causative dermatophyte. It primarily affects children between three and 14 years of age (prepubertal). Posterior cervical lymphadenopathy is often present; it may serve as a clinical pearl in differentiating tinea capitis from other inflammatory disorders involving the scalp [1]. Mycological examinations are considered to be the gold standard diagnostic methods of TC. The samples of hairs, scalp and scales are examined directly by microscope as well as cultured on Sabouraud dextrose agar. However, fungal culture is time-consuming and usually requires two to four weeks for results. A Wood's lamp examination could be useful in some cases in which the causative agent shows fluorescence. Hairs infected by *Microsporum canis, Microsporum audouinii, Microsporum rivalieri, and Microsporum ferrugineum* fluorescence a bright green to yellow-green color [2]. Comma hairs and bar code-like hairs are the classic dermoscopic findings of TC [3].

Treatment for TC relies on the use of systemic antifungal agents since topical agents cannot penetrate the hair shaft. Griseofulvin is known as the gold standard therapy for TC. The treatment with griseofulvin should last four to eight weeks (minimally) until three to six months [4]. Adjuvant therapy with selenium sulfide (1% and 2.5%), zinc pyrithione (1% and 2%), povidone-iodine (2.5%), and ketoconazole (2%) help eradicate dermatophytes from the scalp. Adjunctive use of these shampoos is recommended two to four times weekly for two–four weeks. The thrice weekly use of ketoconazole 2% shampoo or selenium sulfide 2.5% by all household members also reduces transmission by decreasing the shedding of spores. Oral glucocorticoids may reduce the incidence of scarring associated with markedly inflammatory varieties of TC. Although there is no consistent evidence for improved cure rates with use of oral glucocorticoids, they appear to relieve pain and swelling associated with infections. The usual regimen is prednisone 1–2 mg/kg each morning during the first week of therapy [5].

Key Points
- Kerion represents the inflammatory form of tinea capitis
- Oral corticosteroids for kerion may reduce inflammation response and the risk of permanent scarring alopecia

References

1. Zaraa A, Hawilo A, Aounallah S, El Trojjet D, Euch MM, et al. Inflammatory tinea capitis: a 12-year study and a review of the literature. Mycoses. 2013;56:110–6.
2. Leung AKC, Hon KL, Leong KF, Barankin B, Lam JM. Tinea capitis: an updated review. Recent Patents Inflamm Allergy Drug Discov. 2020;14:58–68.
3. Brasileiro A, Campos S, Cabete J, Galhardas C, Lencastre A, Serrao V. Trichoscopy as an additional tool for the differential diagnosis of tinea capitis: a prospective clinical study. Br J Dermatol. 2016;175:208–9.
4. Nakagawa H, Nishihara M, Nakamura T. Kerion and tinea capitis. IDCases. 2018;14:e00418.
5. Fuller LC, Barton RC, Mohd Mustapa MF, et al. British Association of Dermatologists' guidelines for the management for tinea capitis 2014. Br J Dermatol. 2014;171:454–63.

Chapter 28
An Inflammatory Scalp Lesion with Hair Loss

Amr M. Ammar, Shady M. Ibrahim, and Mohamed L. Elsaie

A 10-year-old child presented with a localized area of hair loss.

A physical examination revealed a few pustules overlying erythematous plaque with incomplete alopecia on occipital region (Fig. 28.1).

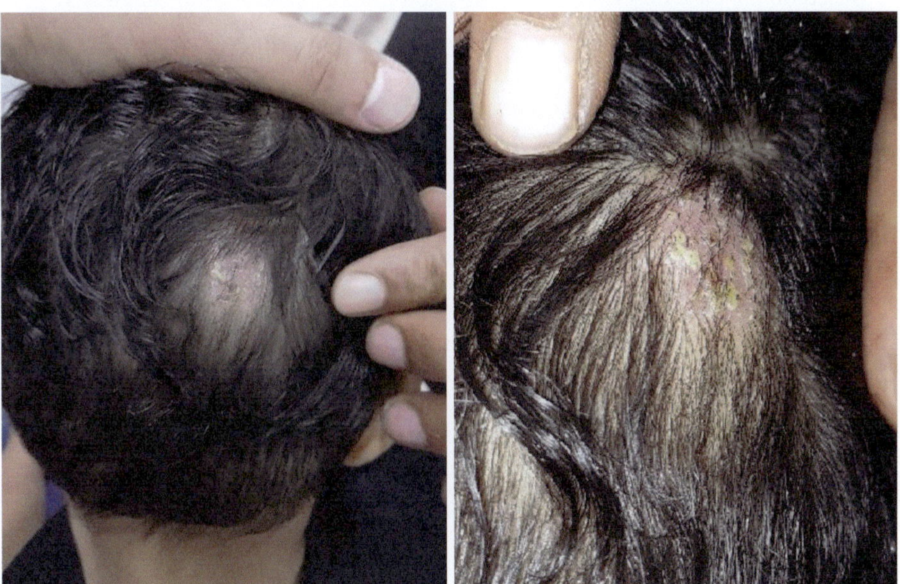

Fig. 28.1 An erythematous plaque with pustules and incomplete hair loss on the occipital region

A. M. Ammar · S. M. Ibrahim
Department of Dermatology and Venerology, Al-Azhar University, Cairo, Egypt

M. L. Elsaie (✉)
Department of Dermatology and Venereology, National Research Center, Cairo, Egypt

© The Author(s), under exclusive license to Springer Nature Switzerland AG 2022
A. Waśkiel-Burnat et al. (eds.), *Clinical Cases in Hair Disorders*, Clinical Cases in Dermatology, https://doi.org/10.1007/978-3-030-93423-1_28

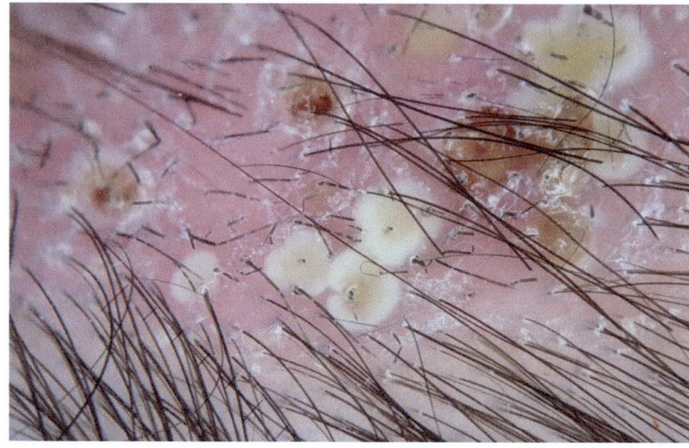

Fig. 28.2 Dermoscopy shows a few pustules overlying erythematous background, white sheaths around the proximal hair shafts and Morse code-like hairs

Dermoscophy showed a few pustules overlying erythematous background, white sheaths around the proximal hair shafts, Morse code-like hairs, broken and dystrophic hairs, i hairs and crusts (Figs. 28.2 and 28.3).

Based on the case description and the photographs, what is your diagnosis?

Differential Diagnoses

1. Alopecia areata.
2. Kerion (inflammatory tinea capitis).
3. Discoid lupus erythematosus.
4. Dissecting cellulitis of the scalp.

Diagnosis

Kerion (inflammatory tinea capitis).

Discussion

Tinea capitis is a common infection of the scalp hair caused by dermatophyte fungi and occurring predominantly in children. Its clinical manifestations range from mild scaling with little hair loss to large inflammatory and pustular plaques with extensive alopecia. Although prevalent in many countries in the early twentieth century, it was brought under effective control in Europe and North America after the introduction of griseofulvin and concerted public health interventions, whereas it

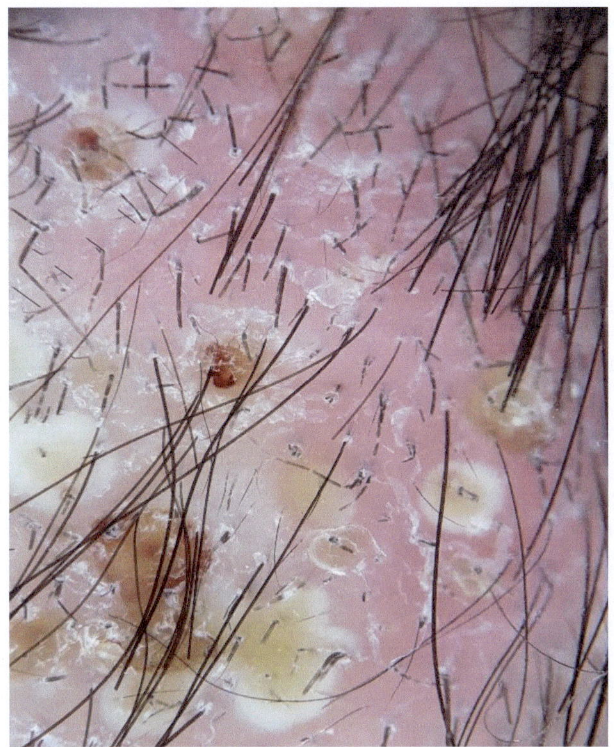

Fig. 28.3 Dermoscopy with the presence of Morse code-like hairs, pustules, broken and dystrophic hairs, i hairs and crusts

remained endemic in other regions. However, over the last 10–20 years, this situation has changed with the spread of organisms, in particular Trichophyton tonsurans, in the Americas, Europe and Africa [1].

There is a spectrum of clinical reactions in tinea capitis that also reflects the pathological changes. In some patients, there is a pronounced inflammatory reaction, a feature often seen in zoophilic infections or those spread from animals to human; by contrast in others, particularly those with anthropophilic dermatophytosis spread from human to human, lesions are often non-inflammatory and persistent. It is still not clear whether this reflects the level of immunological responsiveness to these infections and the vast majority of those affected have no underlying predisposing illness [2].

Hair penetration by dermatophytes involves the production of proteases, some of which are inducible in the presence of amino acid residues as well as disruption of intercellular junctions due to hyphal turgor pressure. Dermatophytes produce a variety of proteolytic enzymes, which work in acid, alkali or neutral environments [3].

Many species of dermatophytes are capable of invading hair shafts, but some (e.g. Trichophyton tonsurans, Trichophyton schoenleinii and Trichophyton violaceum) have a predilection for this pattern of infection, whereas Epidermophyton floccosum and Trichophyton concentricum do not cause tinea capitis [1, 4]. The clinical appearance of ringworm of the scalp is variable, depending on the type of hair invasion, the level of host resistance and the degree of inflammatory host response. Most affected patients are children for 6 months to 10–12 years of age.

The most severe pattern of reaction is known as a kerion. It is a painful, inflammatory mass in which those hairs that remain are loose. Follicles discharge pus. The affected area is usually limited, but occasionally, a large confluent may involve much of the scalp. Lymphadenopathy is frequent. This reaction is usually caused by one of the zoophilic species, typically Trichophyton verrucosum or Trichophyton mentagrophytes, but occasionally, anthropophilic infections may suddenly become inflammatory and develop into kerions. Generally, however, pustule formation represents an inflammatory response to the fungus itself rather than a secondary bacterial infection. If secondary bacterial infection occurs, it is usually present under crusts covering the inflammatory mass and removal of these is an important part of management. Another adaptation of a diagnostic technique widely used in dermatology has been to employ the dermatoscope for close inspection of the scalp [5]. Although, not as yet subject to comparative study, there are visual features of the scalp on infected areas that may be distinctive for different organisms. For instance, in infections caused by Trichophyton tonsurans, the infected areas showed multiple comma-shaped hairs, whereas with Microsporum canis, dermoscopy shows dystrophic and elbow-shaped hairs, and in addition, there are different height levels of broken hair [6].

Topical antifungal therapy has little place in the management of tinea capitis except as an adjunct to oral therapy. There is evidence that final relapse rates of infection following topical therapy are high, although the clinical appearances and itching may initially improve. Treatment for tinea capitis relies on the use of terbinafine, itraconazole, griseofulvin and fluconazole [1, 7].

There is no clinical evidence to support the use of other oral antifungals, including the newer azoles such as voriconazole or posaconazole. Griseofulvin was the first effective drug used of the treatment of tinea capitis and is still widely used in resource-poor settings as it remains effective. It is useful particularly for Microsporum infections, but it is not available in paediatric form (liquid or small tablet sizes) in many countries. Although massive single-dose therapy with griseofulvin and intermittent dose regimens (25 mg/kg twice a week) have had some success, in general, conventional daily therapy is advisable (10–15 mg/kg). In small-spored ectothrix infections, griseofulvin for at least six weeks is usually adequate. In some infections such as those caused by Trichophyton tonsurans and Trichophyton schoenleinii infections, much longer courses and sometimes higher dosage (20 mg/kg/day) of griseofulvin therapy may be needed.

Control of tinea capitis is not impossible, and with current understanding of the immunology and host susceptibility, including the latest findings of specific CARD 9 gene mutations associated with widespread deep dermatophytosis [8].

Key Points
- Tinea capitis is a common infection of the scalp hair caused by dermatophyte fungi and occurring predominantly in children
- The most severe pattern of reaction is known as a kerion. It is a painful, inflammatory mass in which those hairs that remain are loose
- Topical antifungal therapy has little place in the management of tinea capitis except as an adjunct to oral therapy

References

1. Elewski BE. Tinea capitis: a current perspective. J Am Acad Dermatol. 2000;42:1–20.
2. Zurita J, Hay RJ. The adherence of dermatophyte microconidia and arthroconidia to human keratinocytes in vitro. J Invest Dermatol. 1987;89:529–34.
3. Sriranganadane D, Waridel P, Salamin K, et al. Identification of novel secreted proteases during extracellular proteolysis by dermatophytes at acidic pH. Proteomics. 2011;11:4422–33.
4. Fuller LC, Child FC, Higgins EM. Tinea capitis in Southeast London: an outbreak of Trichophyton tonsurans infection. Br J Dermatol. 1997;136:139–45.
5. Brasileiro A, Campos S, Cabete J, et al. Trichoscopy as an additional tool for the differential diagnosis of tinea capitis. Br J Dermatol. 2016;175(1):208–9. https://doi.org/10.1111/bjd.14413.
6. Schechtman RC, Silva ND, Quaresma MV, et al. Dermatoscopic findings as a complementary tool in the differential diagnosis of the etiological agent of tinea capitis. Ann Bras Dermatol. 2015;90(Suppl 1):13–5.
7. Fuller CF, Barton RC, Mohd Mustapa MF, et al. British Association of Dermatologists' guidelines for the management of tinea capitis 2014. Br J Dermatol. 2014;171:454–63.
8. Lanternier F, Pathan S, Vincent QB, et al. Deep dermatophytosis and inherited CARD9 deficiency. N Engl J Med. 2013;369:1704–14.

Chapter 29
An Localized Alopecia on the Scalp

Amr M. Ammar, Shady M. Ibrahim, and Mohamed L. Elsaie

A 52-year-old female patient presented with an localized area of incomplete alopecia.

A physical examination revealed ill-defined patchy areas of incomplete alopecia (Fig. 29.1).

Dermoscopy showed localized ivory white structureless areas of alopecia with the absence of follicular openings. The remaining follicles showed perifollicular scaling and violaceous structureless areas (Fig. 29.2).

Based on the case description, clinical and dermoscopic photographs, what is your diagnosis?

Differential Diagnoses

1. Alopecia areata.
2. Lichen planopilaris.
3. Discoid lupus erythematosus.
4. Dissecting cellulitis.

A. M. Ammar · S. M. Ibrahim
Department of Dermatology and Venerology, Al-Azhar University, Cairo, Egypt

M. L. Elsaie (✉)
Department of Dermatology and Venereology, National Research Center, Cairo, Egypt

A. Waśkiel-Burnat et al. (eds.), *Clinical Cases in Hair Disorders*, Clinical Cases in Dermatology, https://doi.org/10.1007/978-3-030-93423-1_29

Fig. 29.1 In ill-defined patchy areas of incomplete alopecia

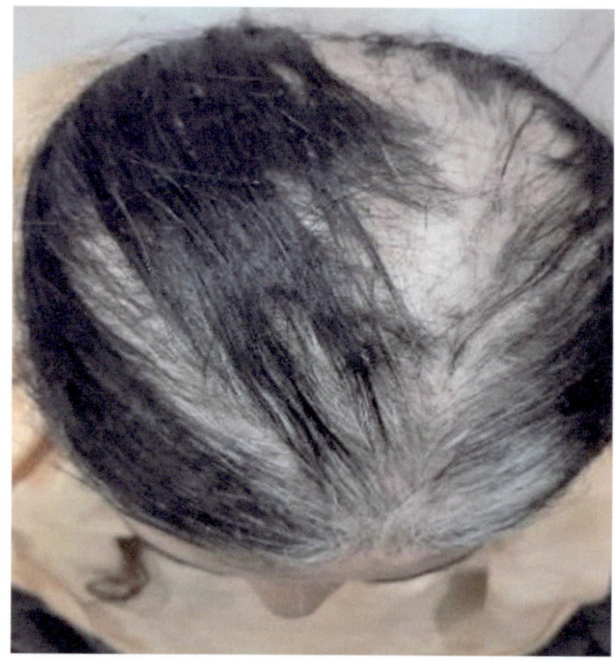

Fig. 29.2 Dermoscopy shows localized ivory white structureless areas of alopecia with the absence of follicular openings. The remaining follicles showed perifollicular scaling and violaceous structureless areas

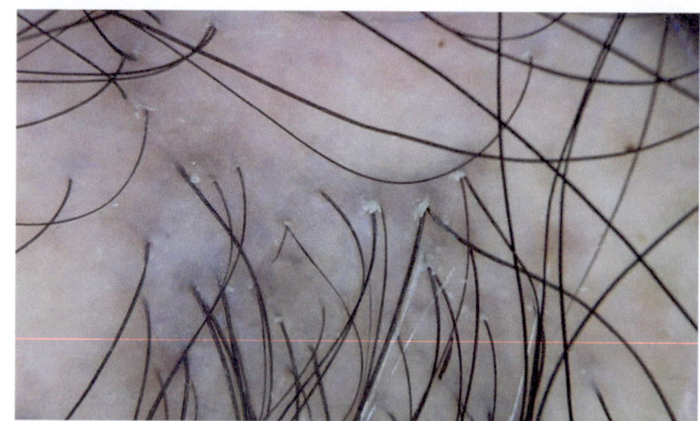

Diagnosis

Lichen planopilaris.

Discussion

Lichen planopilaris (LPP) is a primary cicatricial alopecia caused by chronic lymphocytic inflammation around the upper portion of the hair follicle. The origin of LPP, and the other primary cicatricial alopecias, remains poorly understood, but they all have in common a targeted folliculocentric attack, which leads to irreversible follicular destruction and permanent hair loss [1].

LPP usually presents as irregular patchy hair loss, with loss of follicular ostia, a hallmark of all cicatricial alopecias. Less commonly the hair loss is diffuse rather than patchy. Perifollicular erythema and perifollicular scale are typically present at the periphery of active lesions. Cutaneous lichen planus may develop before, during, or after the onset of LPP. Oral and genital lesions may also occur. Many patients have a history of scalp scaling, often considered seborrheic dermatitis, for many years before the diagnosis of LPP. Active, untreated LPP is often intensely symptomatic with severe pruritus, pain, tenderness, and burning [2].

Diagnosis of LPP always requires clinicopathological correlation and cannot be made by the above clinical signs and symptoms alone. At least one four mm deep punch biopsy specimen down to subcutaneous fat is submitted for horizontal sectioning and hematoxylin-eosin staining. Compared with vertical sectioning where three–four follicles may be acquired, horizontal sectioning allows up to 30 follicles to be examined. The biopsy site is an active, symptomatic hair-bearing area with perifollicular erythema and perifollicular scale, located at the margin of a bare patch, with a positive anagen pull test result when possible [1, 2].

The most common trichoscopic features of classic lichen planopilaris include the absence of follicular openings, perifollicular scaling and white cicatricial areas. Other common trichoscopic findings are perifollicular erythema, milky-red areas, classic white and blue-grey dots [3–5]. Perifollicular erythema and white cicatricial areas are associated with disease severity [3].

Key Points
- Lichen planopilaris usually presents as irregular patchy hair loss, with loss of follicular ostia
- Diagnosis of lichen planopilaris always requires clinicopathological correlation and cannot be made by the clinical signs and symptoms alone

References

1. Templeton S, Solomon A. Scarring alopecia: a classification based on microscopic criteria. J Cutan Pathol. 1994;21:97–109.
2. Tan E, Martinka M, Ball N, Shapiro J. Primary cicatricial alopecias: clinicopathology of 112 cases. J Am Acad Dermatol. 2004;50:25–32.
3. Rakowska A, Slowinska M, Kowalska-Oledzka E, Warszawik O, Czuwara J, Olszewska M, Rudnicka L. Trichoscopy of cicatricial alopecia. J Drugs Dermatol. 2012;11(6):753–8.
4. Kossard S, Zagarella S. Spotted cicatricial alopecia in dark skin. A dermoscopic clue to fibrous tracts. Australas J Dermatol. 1993;34:49–51.
5. Duque-Estrada B, Tamler C, Sodré CT, Barcaui CB, Pereira FB. Dermoscopy patterns of cicatricial alopecia resulting from discoid lupus erythematosus and lichen planopilaris. An Bras Dermatol. 2010;85:179–83.

Chapter 30
Patches of Non-scarring Alopecia in a 22-Year-Old Male

Ioana-Simona Dinu, Emanuela-Domnica Boieriu, Iulia-Elena Negulet, Alexandra-Irina Butacu, and George-Sorin Tiplica

A 22-year-old male presented to the Dermatological Department with well-defined patches of non-scarring alopecia without inflammation signs. The hair loss started one year ago as small patches and gradually increased in size and number. Family history and personal medical history were negative. No history of drug intake as well as photosensitivity was reported.

A physical examination revealed multiple well-defined patches of non-scarring alopecia, oval in shape, with no associated skin changes, located on the occipital and both temporal regions (Fig. 30.1). Dermoscopy showed black dots and exclamation mark hairs. Patches of alopecia were not observed within the eyelashes, eyebrows or other body regions. Nails were not affected.

A direct mycological test with potassium hydroxide showed no fungal elements.

Laboratory investigations were normal. No autoimmune markers were identified, such as antinuclear antibodies, anti-ds DNA antibodies, anti-thyroperoxidase antibodies; the complement and its fractions (C3, C4) were normal. Syphilis serology was negative.

Based on the case description and the photographs, what is your diagnosis?

Differential Diagnoses

1. Alopecia areata.
2. Syphilitic alopecia.
3. Tinea capitis.
4. Discoid lupus erythematosus.

I.-S. Dinu · E.-D. Boieriu · I.-E. Negulet · A.-I. Butacu (✉) · G.-S. Tiplica
2nd Department of Dermatology, Colentina Clinical Hospital, "Carol Davila" University of Medicine and Pharmacy, Bucharest, Romania

A. Waśkiel-Burnat et al. (eds.), *Clinical Cases in Hair Disorders*, Clinical Cases in Dermatology, https://doi.org/10.1007/978-3-030-93423-1_30

Fig. 30.1 Well-demarcated patches of alopecia on the occipital region of the scalp

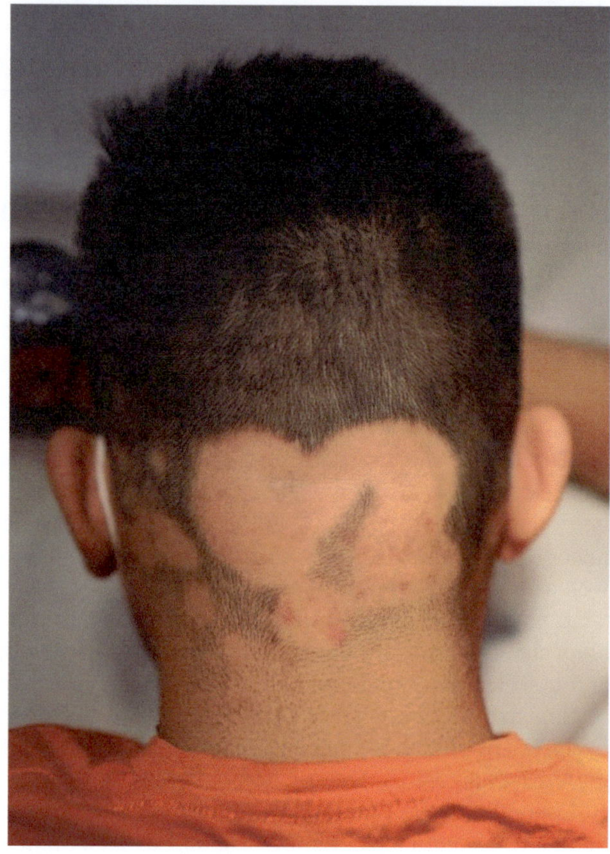

Diagnosis

Alopecia areata.

Discussion

Alopecia areata is an autoimmune, non-scarring hair loss disorder, being one of the most common cause of hair loss [1]. In the general population, there is a 2% risk of developing this condition during lifetime [2]. The disease can be diagnosed at any age [3]. Alopecia areata may evolve into alopecia totalis and *alopecia universalis* [1]. The triggers that precipitate the autoimmune reaction are unknown, even though infections, stress and drugs could be involved. As a result of the immune response, the hair follicle prematurely enters the catagen phase [2]. The clinical examination reveals round, smooth, well demarcated patches of alopecia, with normal skin within the affected sites. At the margins of the lesions, exclamation mark hairs can be observed [3]. Black dots could also be observed through dermoscopy. The diagnosis is based on clinical findings. Trichoscopy and skin biopsy further support the diagnosis [1].

Syphilitic alopecia also called alopecia areolaris represents a clinical sign that occurs in only 4% of cases of syphilis, being most frequent in secondary syphilis [4]. It is caused by the inflammation of the hair follicles induced by *Treponema pallidum*. The condition can be classified as patchy, which is the most common form, or diffuse [5]. The clinical examination reveals patches of non-scarring alopecia of different size, without signs of inflammation. The margins of the lesions are not well defined, and the areas of alopecia are not completely hairless with a "moth-eaten pattern". This disease involves especially the parieto-occipital region, probably because important blood supply exists in this region. The diagnosis is established on clinical findings and laboratory tests, such as syphilis serology or immunohistochemistry [4]. The immunohistochemical study is considered to have the greatest sensitivity, as it detects spirochetes in the inflammatory infiltrate [5].

Tinea capitis is a fungal infection of hair and scalp typically caused by *Trichophyton* and *Microsporum* species that most often presents with pruritic, scaling areas of hair loss [6]. The infection is often transmitted through direct contact with an infected human or animal or through contact with a contaminated object. Children, particularly prepubertal children, are most likely to develop tinea capitis [7]. Inflammation and cervical lymphadenopathy may also be present. Tinea capitis should always be considered in children presenting with patchy hair loss. The disease is characterized the presence of a single scaly patch of alopecia in case of ectothrix tinea capitis and by multiple, polygonal patches of alopecia with follicular black dots in case of endothrix tinea capitis. In case of kerion celsi, the lesions consits of a inflammatory, painful mass with nodules, plaques, purulent discharge and hair loss. Tinea capitis can be diagnosed based upon the physical examination, laboratory investigations such as direct mycological test with potassium hydroxide, fungal culture or PCR techniques which can detect fungal DNA. On Wood's lamp examination, a yellow-green fluorescence may be detected, depending on the causative organism [8].

Chronic cutaneous lupus erythematosus includes several clinical types, such as discoid lupus erythematosus, chilblain lupus or lupus tumidus. Discoid lupus erythematosus is described as a chronic, scarring, atrophy-producing, photosensitive dermatosis. It may occur at any age, but it is most frequently diagnosed in persons aged 20–40 years [9]. Discoid lupus erythematosus most often involves the face, scalp and neck but may also occur on the ears. The scalp involvement is the most common presentation of discoid lupus erythematosus [10]. Cicatricial alopecia may be the result of discoid lupus erythematosus, being characterized by permanent destruction of hair follicles. Hair loss is usually patchy and there is loss of follicular orifices in sites of alopecia. Erythema, scale, atrophy and pigmentary changes are commonly seen in the center of discoid lesions rather than at the periphery of hair loss. Discoid lupus erythematosus located on the scalp may be itchy, associated with burning, stinging sensation or may be asymptomatic. Non-scarring diffuse alopecia

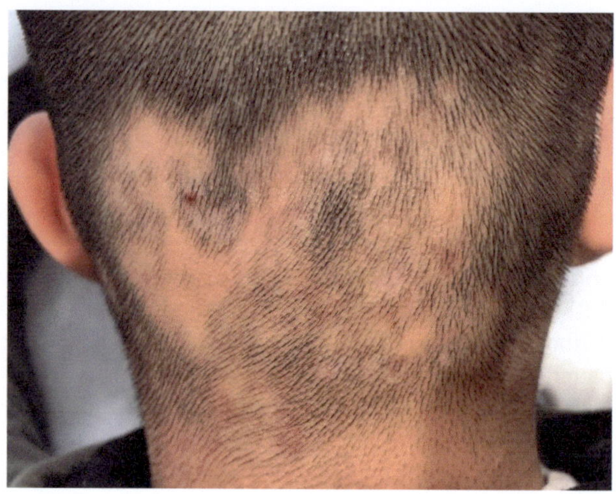

Fig. 30.2 Partial hair regrowth on the occipital region of the scalp after five months of treatment

can appear in patients with systemic lupus erythematosus. The diagnosis of systemic lupus erythematosus is generally based on clinical and laboratory criteria [10]. Skin biopsy and direct immunofluorescence examination of tissue samples may also be beneficial to establishing the diagnosis [9].

In the presented patient, on the basis of clinical examination and laboratory investigations, the diagnosis of alopecia areata was established. Treatment with intralesional triamcinolone acetonide (5 mg/ml) every four weeks was initiated with significant improvement five months after treatment initiation (complete hair regrowth on the right temporal region and partial regrowth on the occipital and left temporal region) (Fig. 30.2).

Key Points
- Alopecia areata represents an autoimmune, non-scarring hair loss disorder
- Alopecia areata may occur at any age
- Alopecia areata may evolve into alopecia totalis and *alopecia universalis*
- The clinical examination reveals round, smooth, well demarcated patches of alopecia, with normal skin on the affected sites
- The diagnosis of alopecia areata is usually based on clinical findings

References

1. Pratt CH, King LE Jr, Messenger AG, Christiano AM, Sundberg JP. Alopecia areata. Nat Rev Dis Primers. 2017;3:17011. https://doi.org/10.1038/nrdp.2017.11.
2. Lepe K, Zito PM. Alopecia Areata. 2020 Sep 29. In: StatPearls [Internet]. Treasure Island, FL: StatPearls Publishing; 2020 Jan.

3. Darwin E, Hirt PA, Fertig R, Doliner B, Delcanto G, Jimenez JJ. Alopecia Areata: review of epidemiology, clinical features, pathogenesis, and new treatment options. Int J Trichology. 2018;10(2):51–60. https://doi.org/10.4103/ijt.ijt_99_17.
4. Hernández-Bel P, Unamuno B, Sánchez-Carazo JL, Febrer I, Alegre V. Syphilitic alopecia: a report of 5 cases and a review of the literature. Actas Dermosifiliogr. 2013;104(6):512–7. https://doi.org/10.1016/j.ad.2012.02.009.
5. Bernárdez C, Molina-Ruiz AM, Requena L. Histologic features of alopecias-part I: non-scarring alopecias. Actas Dermosifiliogr. 2015;106(3):158–67. https://doi.org/10.1016/j.ad.2014.07.006.
6. Leung AKC, Hon KL, Leong KF, Barankin B, Lam JM. Tinea capitis: an updated review. Recent Patents Inflamm Allergy Drug Discov. 2020;14(1):58–68. https://doi.org/10.2174/1872213X14666200106145624.
7. Mirmirani P, Tucker LY. Epidemiologic trends in pediatric tinea capitis: a population-based study from Kaiser Permanente Northern California. J Am Acad Dermatol. 2013;69(6):916–21. https://doi.org/10.1016/j.jaad.2013.08.031.
8. Petrucelli MF, Abreu MH, Cantelli BAM, Segura GG, Nishimura FG, Bitencourt TA, Marins M, Fachin AL. Epidemiology and diagnostic perspectives of dermatophytoses. J Fungi (Basel). 2020;6(4):310. https://doi.org/10.3390/jof6040310.
9. Hordinsky M. Cicatricial alopecia: discoid lupus erythematosus. Dermatol Ther. 2008;21(4):245–8. https://doi.org/10.1111/j.1529-8019.2008.00205.x.
10. Concha JSS, Werth VP. Alopecias in lupus erythematosus. Lupus Sci Med. 2018;5(1):e000291. https://doi.org/10.1136/lupus-2018-000291.

Chapter 31
Patchy Atypical Hair Loss in an Infant

Amr M. Ammar, Shady M. Ibrahim, and Mohamed L. Elsaie

A three-month-old male infant presented with localized area of hair loss of two-month duration.

A physical examination revealed localized area of incomplete alopecia on the vertex (Fig. 31.1).

Dermoscopy showed yellow amorphous structureless areas, Z hairs, corkscrew hairs, coma hairs, black dots and broken hairs in addition to diffuse erythema (Figs. 31.2 and 31.3).

Based on the case description and the photographs, what is your diagnosis?

Differential Diagnoses

1. Alopecia areata.
2. Tinea capitis (Inflammatory type).
3. Aplasia cutis congenita.
4. Nevus sebaceus of Jadassohn.

Diagnosis

Tinea capitis (Inflammatory type).

A. M. Ammar · S. M. Ibrahim
Department of Dermatology and Venerology, Al-Azhar University, Cairo, Egypt

M. L. Elsaie (✉)
Department of Dermatology and Venercology, National Research Center, Cairo, Egypt

© The Author(s), under exclusive license to Springer Nature Switzerland AG 2022
A. Waśkiel-Burnat et al. (eds.), *Clinical Cases in Hair Disorders*, Clinical Cases in Dermatology, https://doi.org/10.1007/978-3-030-93423-1_31

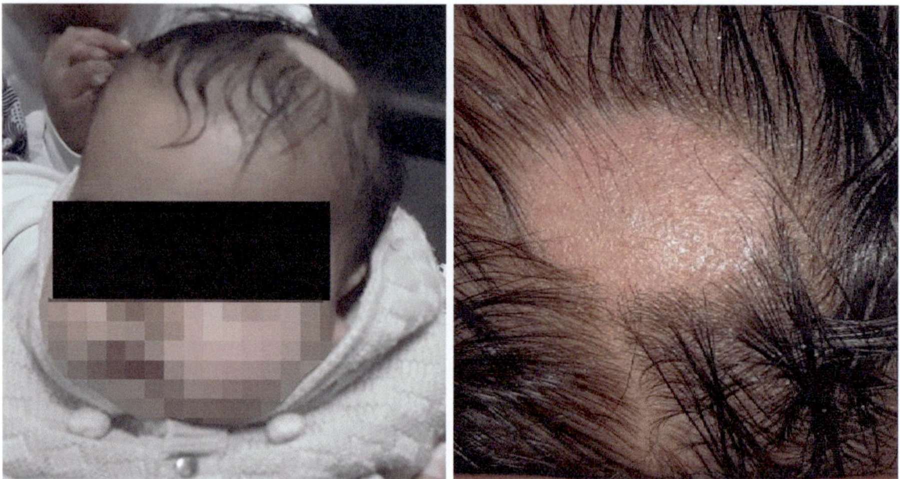

Fig. 31.1 A three-month-old male infant with localized area of incomplete alopecia on the vertex

Fig. 31.2 Dermoscopy shows Z hairs, corkscrew hairs, coma hairs, scaling on erythematous background

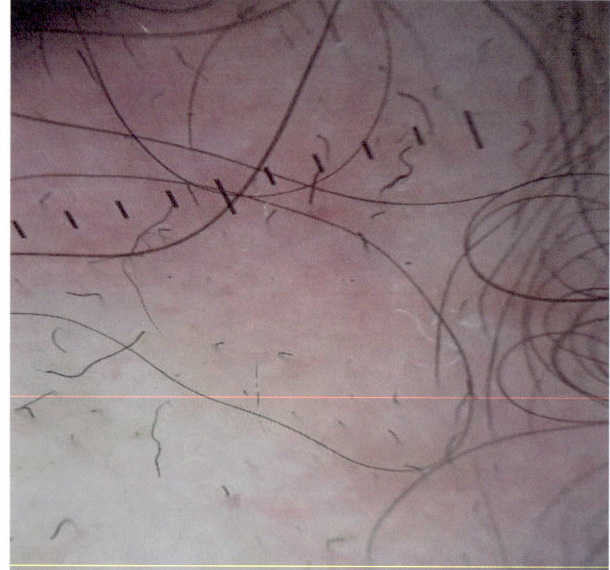

Discussion

Tinea capitis (TC) is a fungal infection of the scalp and the surrounding skin due to dermatophytes such as *Microsporum* spp. and *Trichophyton* spp. [1, 2]. It is a predominantly dermatophyte infection in children three to seven years of age and it is rare in infants in the first year of life [3, 4].

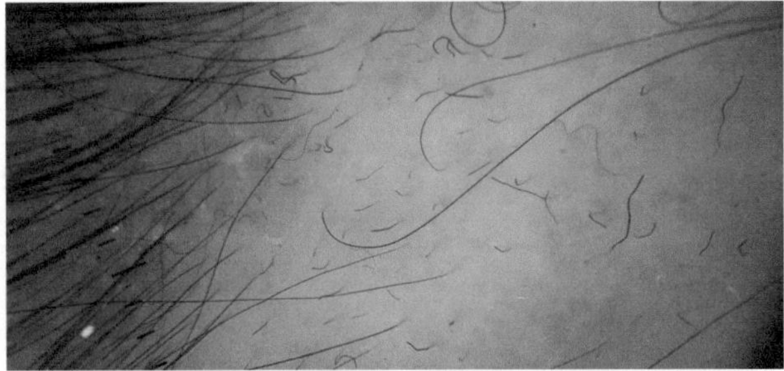

Fig. 31.3 Dermoscopy shows amorphous structureless areas, Z hairs, corkscrew hairs, coma hairs, black dots and broken hairs in addition to diffuse erythema

Epidemiology of TC can be related to geographical location and social, cultural and nutritional factors: in infants, across Europe and the *Mediterranean* basin, Microsporum canis remains the most common organism responsible for TC, with prevalence ranges between 0.23 and 2.6%. *Trichophyton tonsurans* is reported as accounting for 50–90% of dermatophyte scalp isolates in the UK and the USA. In addition, *Trichophyton tonsurans* has spread to both South America and West Africa. *Trichophyton violaceum* is the most common in Greece and Belgium [5–8].

Although the incidence of TC in infants is low, sometimes it is misdiagnosed and underreported. Differential diagnosis for TC includes seborrheic dermatitis, atopic dermatitis, neonatal lupus, Langerhans cell histiocytosis, and syphilis. TC should be suspected in a child with alopecia, pruritus and/or persistent desquamation and thinning hair. The scalp lesion should be investigated from a mycological point of view [6, 9, 10].

The drug of choice for the treatment of TC in children is griseofulvin. Therapy should lasts six to 12 weeks or until the patient tests are negative for fungi (light microscopy and culture). The long period of treatment required with griseofulvin is a significant disadvantage and leads to reduced compliance [8]. Other oral antifungals, specifically fluconazole, itraconazole, ketoconazole, and terbinafine are available and give the advantage of good safety and efficacy profiles, and shorter required duration of treatment of TC caused by *Trichophyton* and *Microsporum* [8].

Key Points
- Tinea capitis is a common infection of the scalp hair caused by dermatophyte fungi and occurring predominantly in children
- The drug of choice for the treatment of tinea capitis in children is griseofulvin
- Topical antifungal therapy has little place in the management of tinea capitis except as an adjunct to oral therapy

References

1. Kundu D, Mandal L, Sen G. Prevalence of tinea capitis in school going children in Kolkata, West Bengal. J Nat Sci Biol Med. 2012;3:152–5.
2. Farooqi M, Tabassum S, Rizvi DA, Rahman A, Rehanuddin AS, Mahar SA. Clinical types of tinea capitis and species identification in children: an experience from tertiary care centres of Karachi, Pakistan. J Pak Med Assoc. 2014;64:304–8.
3. Michaels BD, Del Rosso JQ. Tinea capitis in infants: recognition, evaluation, and management suggestions. J Clin Aesthet Dermatol. 2012;5:49–59.
4. Adefemi SA, Odeigah LO, Alabi KM. Prevalence of dermatophytosis among primary school children in Oke-Oyi community of Kwara state. Niger J Clin Pract. 2011;14:23–8.
5. Tullio V, Cervetti O, Roana J, Panzone M, Scalas D, Merlino C, Allizond V, Banche G, Mandras N, Cuffini AM. Advances in microbiology, infectious diseases and public health: refractory Trichophyton rubrum infections in Turin, Italy: a problem still present. Adv Exp Med Biol. 2016;901:17–23.
6. Atanasovski M, El Tal AK, Hamzavi F, Mehregan DA. Neonatal dermatophytosis: report of a case and review of the literature. Pediatr Dermatol. 2011;28:185–8.
7. Mashiah J, Kutz A, Ben Ami R, Savion M, Goldberg I, Gan Or T, Zidan O, Sprecher E, Harel A. Tinea capitis outbreak among paediatric refugee population, an evolving healthcare challenge. Mycoses. 2016;59:553–7.
8. Bennassar A, Grimalt R. Management of tinea capitis in childhood. Clin Cosmet Investig Dermatol. 2010;3:89–98.
9. Gilaberte Y, Rezusta A, Gil J, Sáenz-Santamaría MC, Coscojuela C, Navarro M, Zubiri ML, Moles B, Rubio MC. Tinea capitis in infants in their first year of life. Br J Dermatol. 2004;151:886–90.
10. Zampella JG, Kwatra SG, Blanck J, Cohen B. Tinea in tots: cases and literature review of oral antifungal treatment of tinea capitis in children under 2 years of age. J Pediatr. 2017;183:12–8.

Chapter 32
Patchy, Bizarre Hair Loss on the Scalp

Amr M. Ammar, Shady M. Ibrahim, and Mohamed L. Elsaie

A 36-year-old male patient presented to the Department Clinic complaining of multiple areas of hair loss on scalp of three months duration.

A physical examination revealed ill-defined localized multiple areas of hair loss on the vertex and temporal areas (Fig. 32.1).

Dermoscopy showed localized areas of incomplete hair loss with multiple broken hairs at different levels, black dots, mace like hairs, flame hairs, broom fibers and hair powder areata (Figs. 32.2 and 32.3).

Based on the case description and the photographs, what is your diagnosis?

Differential Diagnoses

1. Alopecia areata.
2. Tinea capitis.
3. Trichotillomania.
4. Moth Eaten Alopecia of Syphilis.

A. M. Ammar · S. M. Ibrahim
Department of Dermatology and Venerology, Al-Azhar University, Cairo, Egypt

M. L. Elsaie (✉)
Department of Dermatology and Venereology, National Research Center, Cairo, Egypt

A. Waśkiel-Burnat et al. (eds.), *Clinical Cases in Hair Disorders*, Clinical Cases in Dermatology, https://doi.org/10.1007/978-3-030-93423-1_32

A. M. Ammar et al.

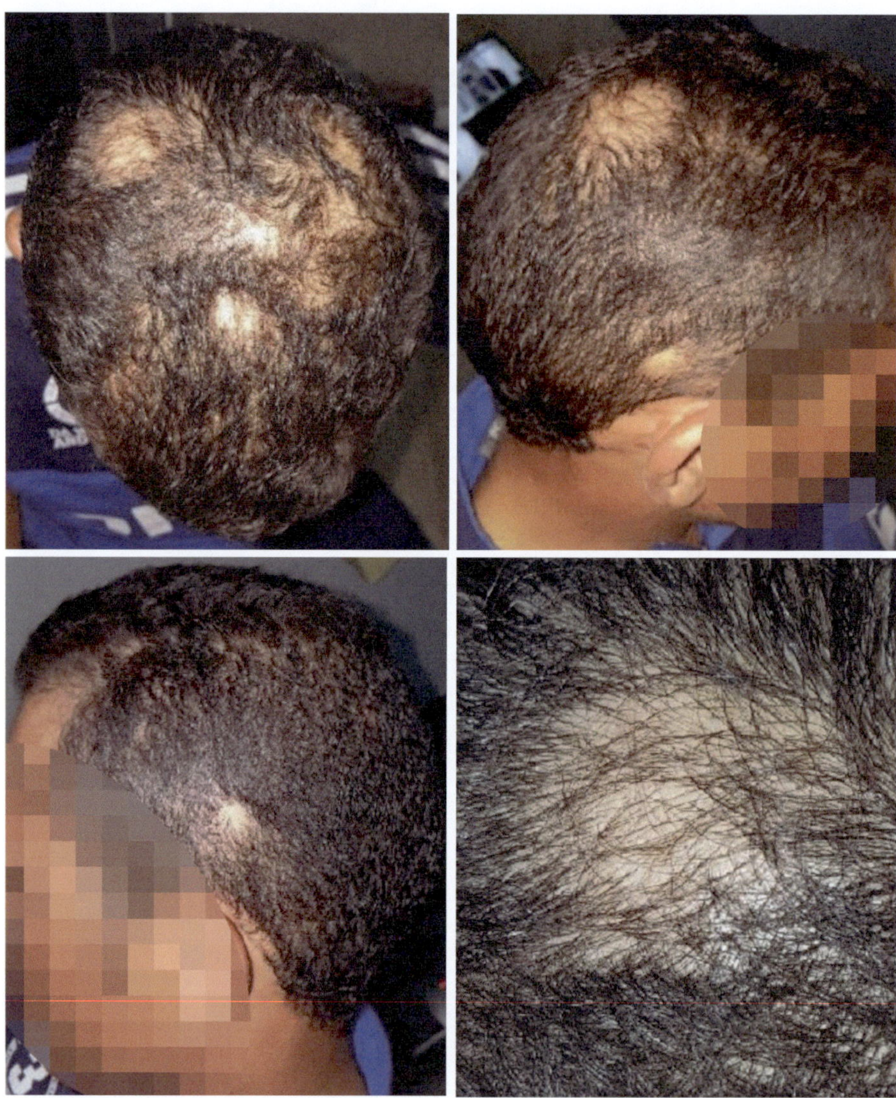

Fig. 32.1 Ill-defined localized multiple areas of hair loss on the vertex and temporal areas

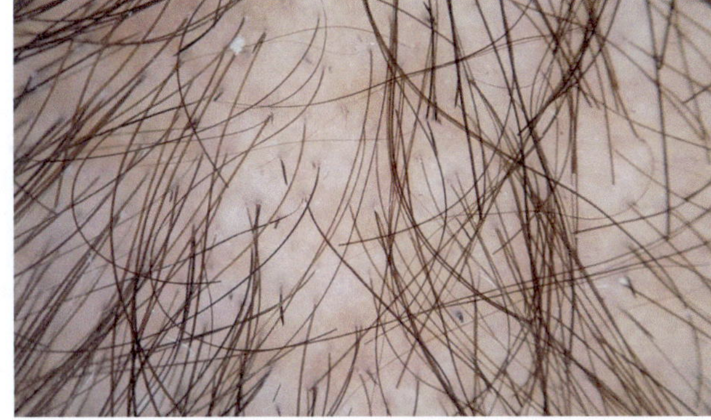

Fig. 32.2 Dermoscopy shows localized areas of incomplete hair loss with multiple broken hairs at different levels, black dots, mace like hairs, flame hairs, broom fibers and hair powder

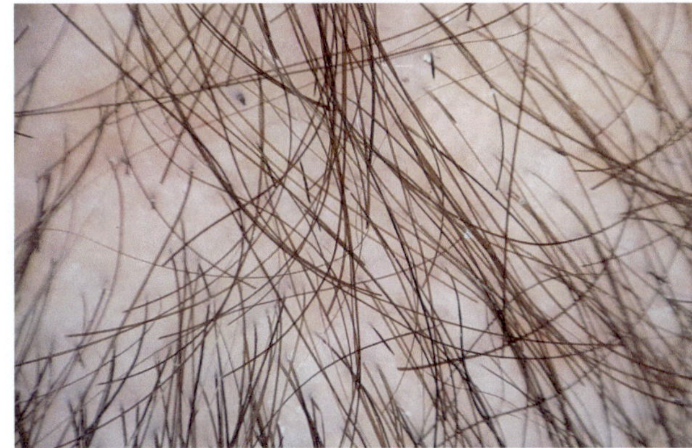

Fig. 32.3 Dermoscopy shows localized areas of incomplete hair loss with multiple broken hairs at different levels, black dots, mace like hairs, flame hairs, broom fibers and hair powder

Diagnosis

Trichotillomania.

Discussion

Trichotillomania is an often debilitating psychiatric condition characterized by recurrent pulling out of one's own hair, leading to hair loss and marked functional impairment [1, 2]. Although discussed in the medical literature for over a century [3], trichotillomania was not officially included as a mental disorder in DSM until 1987, when it was classified as an impulse control disorder not elsewhere classified in DSMIII-R. In DSM-5, trichotillomania was included in the chapter on obsessive-compulsive and related disorders, along with obsessive-compulsive disorder, excoriation disorder, body dysmorphic disorder, and hoarding disorder.

DSM-5 Criteria for Trichotillomaniaa

A. Recurrent pulling out of one's hair, resulting in hair loss, B. Repeated attempts to decrease or stop hair pulling, C. The hair pulling causes clinically significant distress or impairment in social, occupational, or other important areas of functioning, D. The hair pulling or hair loss is not attributable to another medical condition (e.g., a dermatological condition), E. The hair pulling is not better explained by the symptoms of another mental disorder (e.g., attempts to improve a perceived defect or flaw in appearance in body dysmorphic disorder) [4].

The typical age at onset of trichotillomania, usually 10–13 years, is remarkably consistent across studies [5, 6]. This characteristic age at onset appears to be consistent across different cultural settings [7, 8].

In trichotillomania, pulling can be undertaken at any hair-bearing area, but the scalp is the most common site (72.8%) followed by the eyebrows (56.4%) and pubic region (50.7%) [6]. Triggers to pull may be sensory (e.g., hair thickness, length, and location and physical sensations on scalp), emotional (e.g., feeling anxious, bored, tense, or angry), and cognitive (e.g., thoughts about hair and appearance, rigid thinking, and cognitive errors) [5]. In our experience, most individuals report a variety of triggers. Many patients report not being fully aware of their pulling behaviors, at least some of the time—a phenomenon known as "automatic" pulling; "focused" pulling [9].

Trichotillomania may result in unwanted medical consequences. Pulling of hair can lead to skin damage if sharp instruments, such as tweezers or scissors, are used. Over 20% of patients eat hair after pulling it out (trichophagia); a behavior they feel is even more embarrassing than the pulling. In fact, many people with trichotillomania do not divulge this fact until they feel greater trust in the clinician. The ingestion of hair can result in the formation of gastrointestinal hairballs (trichobezoars), which can cause obstructions that may require surgical intervention [10].

In cases of trichotillomania, trichoscopy reveals abnormalities resulting from the stretching and fracture of hair shafts. Fractures may occur at different distances, resulting in irregular black dots, coiled or hook hairs, and hairs with fraying or split ends [11–13]. Black dots (cadaverized hairs) are present inside follicular openings and correspond to the fragmented hair shafts. They are not exclusive of trichotillomania as they are seen also in alopecia areata and tinea capitis. In spite of this, black dots tend to be uniform in size and shape in alopecia areata, whereas in trichotillomania and tinea capitis, a high variability in diameter and shape is found [13]. Flame hairs are semitransparent, wavy, and cone-shaped hair residues that develop as a result of severe mechanical hair pulling. They have been found in alopecia areata, anagen effluvium, and in 25% of affected patients with trichotillomania [11].

Key Points
- Trichotillomania is an often debilitating psychiatric condition characterized by recurrent pulling out of one's own hair, leading to hair loss and marked functional impairment
- In cases of trichotillomania, trichoscopy reveals abnormalities resulting from the stretching and fracture of hair shafts

References

1. Begin with a thorough psychiatric assessment to establish an accurate diagnosis and to assess for co-occurring psychiatric disorders.
2. Conduct a thorough medical evaluation if the patient admits to ingesting hair, to assess for possible gastrointestinal blockage.
3. Provide education about the disorder, including its possible etiologies and the benefits and risks of treatment.
4. Reprinted from American Psychiatric Association: Diagnostic and Statistical Manual of Mental Disorders, Fifth Edition, Arlington, VA: American Psychiatric Association, 2013, p. 251. Copyright 2013, American Psychiatric Association.
5. Christenson GA. Trichotillomania: from prevalence to comorbidity. Psychiatr Times. 1995;12:44–8.
6. Cohen LJ, Stein DJ, Simeon D, et al. Clinical profile, comorbidity, and treatment history in 123 hair pullers: a survey study. J Clin Psychiatry. 1995;56:319–26.
7. Woods DW, Flessner CA, Franklin ME, et al. The Trichotillomania Impact Project (TIP): exploring phenomenology, functional impairment, and treatment utilization. J Clin Psychiatry. 2006;67:1877–88.
8. Duke DC, Keeley ML, Geffken GR, et al. Trichotillomania: a current review. Clin Psychol Rev. 2010;30:181–93.
9. Christenson GA, Mansueto CS. Trichotillomania: descriptive characteristics and phenomenology. In: Stein DJ, Christianson GA, Hollander E, editors. Trichotillomania. Washington, DC: American Psychiatric Press; 1999. p. 1–41.
10. Grant JE, Odlaug BL. Clinical characteristics of trichotillomania with trichophagia. Compr Psychiatry. 2008;49:579–84.
11. Rakowska A, Slowinska M, Olszewska M, Rudnicka L. New trichoscopy findings in trichotillomania: flame hairs, V-sign, hook hairs, hair powder, and tulip hairs. Acta Derm Venereol. 2014;94:303–6.
12. Lee DY, Lee JH, Yang JM, Lee ES. The use of dermoscopy for the diagnosis of trichotillomania. J Eur Acad Dermatol Venereol. 2009;23:731–2.
13. Abraham LS, Torres FN, Azulay-Abulafia L. Dermoscopic clues to distinguish trichotillomania from patchy alopecia areata. An Bras Dermatol. 2010;85:723–6.

Chapter 33
Patterned Hair Loss

Shashank Bhargava and Antonella Tosti

A 47-year-old man presented with patterned symmetric hair loss in centroparietal distribution. The problem started two years back and was slowly progressive. He also complained of itching of the scalp. There was sparing of androgen-independent scalp hair and there were not patches of hair loss. There was no history of any skin lesion else in the body especially over the chest, face and volar aspect of wrist. There was no history of loss eyebrows or any other body hair. He was insisting to undergo hair transplantation (Fig. 33.1).

On general examination, the patient was very much stable. On trichoscopic examination, hair diameter variability and predominance of single hair follicle was noted. Also, we observed loss of follicular openings, perifollicular erythema and perifollicular hyperkeratosis (peripilar casts) (Fig. 33.2).

Based on the case description and the photographs, what is your diagnosis?

Differential Diagnoses

1. Fibrosing alopecia in a pattern distribution.
2. Androgenetic alopecia.
3. Lichen planopilaris.
4. Seborrheic dermatitis.

S. Bhargava (✉)
Department of Dermatology, R. D. Gardi Medical College, Ujjain, Madhya Pradesh, India

A. Tosti
Dr. Philip Frost Department of Dermatology and Cutaneous Surgery, Miller School of Medicine, University of Miami, Coral Gables, FL, USA
e-mail: atosti@med.miami.edu

A. Waśkiel-Burnat et al. (eds.), *Clinical Cases in Hair Disorders*, Clinical Cases
in Dermatology, https://doi.org/10.1007/978-3-030-93423-1_33

Fig. 33.1 Patterned symmetric hair loss in centroparietal distribution with sparing of androgen independent hairs

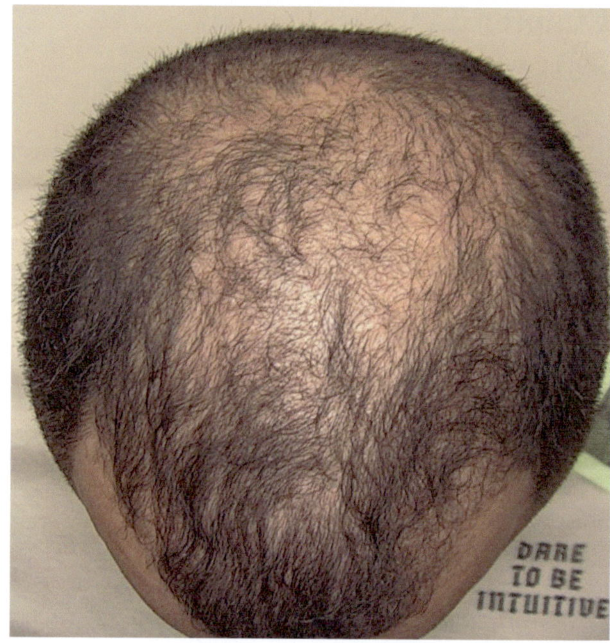

Fig. 33.2 Trichoscopic examination revealing hair shaft variability and peripilar casts

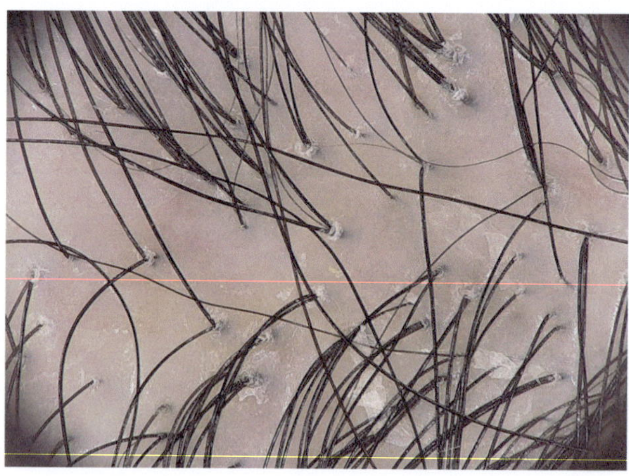

Diagnosis

Fibrosing alopecia in a pattern distribution.

Discussion

In the presented patient, the diagnosis of Fibrosing alopecia in a pattern distribution (FAPD) was made based on clinical and trichoscopic correlation. The diagnosis was confirmed by pathology. FAPD is patterned hair loss involving the androgen dependent sites on the scalp with dermoscopic and/or histopathologic evidence of follicular inflammation and fibrosis without any history of patchy or asymmetric hair loss. It is more common in women where it presents later (postmenopausal) in life as compared to men [1–3]. It is often associated with itching over the scalp and hence it needs to be differentiated from associated seborrheic dermatitis.

The diagnosis is incomplete without trichoscopic and histopathological examination. On trichoscopy, there is peripilar casts/perifollicular hyperkeratosis along with perifollicular erythema and loss of follicular ostia suggesting it to be a variant of lichen planopilaris (LPP). But along with above mentioned findings, there is hair shaft diameter variability with predominance of single hair follicles similar to androgenetic alopecia (AGA) [4, 5]. Further confirmation is made after histopathological examination from the trichoscopic guided site of peripilar casts region [6]. It shows lymphohistiocytic infiltrate around the isthmus and infundibular region of the hair follicle with interface dermatitis; there is also miniaturization of hair follicle with fibrosed follicular tracts [2, 7]. FAPD shares features of both LPP and AGA in the same biopsy specimen. There are chances of coexistent LPP and AGA but with findings of each in different biopsy sample.

It is difficult to understand that why lichenoid tissue reaction particularly occurs over the miniaturized hair follicles in FAPD. There are various theories proposed to understand the pathogenesis of FAPD. One of them suggests the damaged hair follicles may express cytokines that initiate an inflammatory process, another suggests that in immunogenetically susceptible cases a lichenoid tissue reaction can be triggered by an unknown antigenic stimulus on hair follicles that are altered in the genesis of AGA [2, 4].

The treatment should focus on halting the progression of the hair loss. Hence, the medication must reduce the inflammation and also reverse miniaturization. Anti-inflammatory agents like topical steroids and oral antimalarials along with hair promoters like topical minoxidil to thicken the miniaturized hairs are recommended [3, 8, 9]. Other options include anti-androgens like cyproterone and finasteride and topical retinoids can be used to improve the hair loss clinically [2, 3, 10]. None of these medications have been found to work in solo, but always as a combination. These cases are not good candidates for hair transplantation due to potential risk of koebnerization [1].

We started our patient on topical 0.05% clobetasol propionate solution, topical Minoxidil 5% solution and oral minoxidil 1 mg day.

Key Points
- Fibrosing alopecia in a pattern distribution is a form of scarring alopecia with patterned hair loss similar to androgenetic alopecia but with trichoscopic and histopathologic signs of both lichen planopilaris and androgenetic alopecia in the same biopsy specimen
- It is a new entity of patterned hair loss which can be easily missed if dry trichoscopic examination is not performed
- A histopathological examination should always be performed from the trichoscopy guided peripilar casts area
- Hair transplantation should not be performed in these cases due to potential risk of koebnerization and loss of transplanted hair

References

1. Abbasi A, Kamyab-Hesari K, Rabbani R, Mollaee F, Abbasi S. A new subtype of lichen planopilaris affecting vellus hairs and clinically mimicking androgenetic alopecia. Dermatol Surg. 2016;42(10):1174–80.
2. Zinkernagel MS, Trüeb RM. Fibrosing alopecia in a pattern distribution: patterned lichen planopilaris or androgenetic alopecia with a lichenoid tissue reaction pattern? Arch Dermatol. 2000;136(2):205–11.
3. Mardones F, Hott K, Martinez MC. Clinical study of fibrosing alopecia in a pattern distribution in a Latin American population. Int J Dermatol. 2018;57(2):e12–4.
4. Rezende HD, Reis Gavazzoni Dias MF, Trüeb RM. Graft versus host disease presenting as fibrosing alopecia in a pattern distribution: a model for pathophysiological understanding of cicatricial pattern hair loss. Int J Trichology. 2018;10(2):80–3.
5. Vañó-Galván S, Saceda-Corralo D, Blume-Peytavi U, Cucchía J, Dlova NC, Gavazzoni Dias MFR, et al. Frequency of the types of alopecia at twenty-two specialist hair clinics: a multicenter study. Skin Appendage Disord. 2019;5(5):309–15.
6. Griggs J, Trüeb RM, Gavazzoni Dias MFR, Hordinsky M, Tosti A. Fibrosing alopecia in a pattern distribution. J Am Acad Dermatol. 2021;85(6):1557–64. https://doi.org/10.1016/j.jaad.2019.12.056.
7. Teixeira MS, Gavazzoni Dias MFR, Trüeb RM, Rochael MC, Vilar EAG. Fibrosing alopecia in a pattern distribution (FAPD) in 16 African-descent and hispanic female patients: a challenging diagnosis. Skin Appendage Disord. 2019;5(4):211–5.
8. Nic Dhonncha E, Foley CC, Markham T. The role of hydroxychloroquine in the treatment of lichen planopilaris: a retrospective case series and review. Dermatol Ther. 2017;30(3) https://doi.org/10.1111/dth.12463.
9. Stoehr JR, Choi JN, Colavincenzo M, Vanderweil S. Off-label use of topical minoxidil in alopecia: a review. Am J Clin Dermatol. 2019;20(2):237–50.
10. Bergfeld WF. Retinoids and hair growth. J Am Acad Dermatol. 1998;39(2 Pt 3):S86–9.

Chapter 34
Pediculosis Capitis

Ghazala Butt and Muhammad Ahmad

A 14-year-old female presented with nits on the whole scalp for the last two months (Figs. 34.1, 34.2, and 34.3). The scalp was extremely itchy. A detailed history revealed recurrent episodes of the similar condition for the last four years. She tried multiple medications which gave relief only for few weeks and then condition recurred. A physical examination revealed not only nits and lice but also signs of secondary bacterial infection and eczematization on the ears, scalp and eyelids (Fig. 34.4).

Based on the case description and the photographs, what is your diagnosis?

Differential Diagnoses

1. Seborrheic dermatitis.
2. Scabies.
3. Pediculosis capitis.
4. Ezema.

Diagnosis

Pediculosis capitis.

G. Butt (✉)
King Edward Medical University, Lahore, Pakistan

M. Ahmad
Acsthetic Plastic Surgery and FUE Hair Transplant Institute, Islamabad, Pakistan

© The Author(s), under exclusive license to Springer Nature Switzerland AG 2022
A. Waśkiel-Burnat et al. (eds.), *Clinical Cases in Hair Disorders*, Clinical Cases in Dermatology, https://doi.org/10.1007/978-3-030-93423-1_34

Fig. 34.1 Visible lice on hair

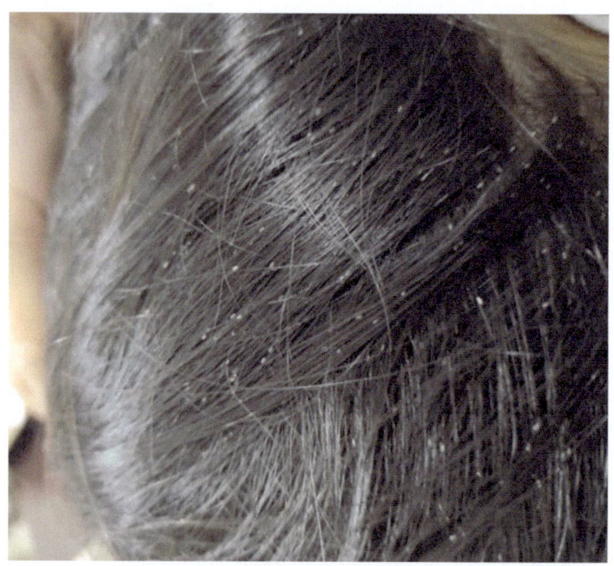

Fig. 34.2 Visible lice on hair

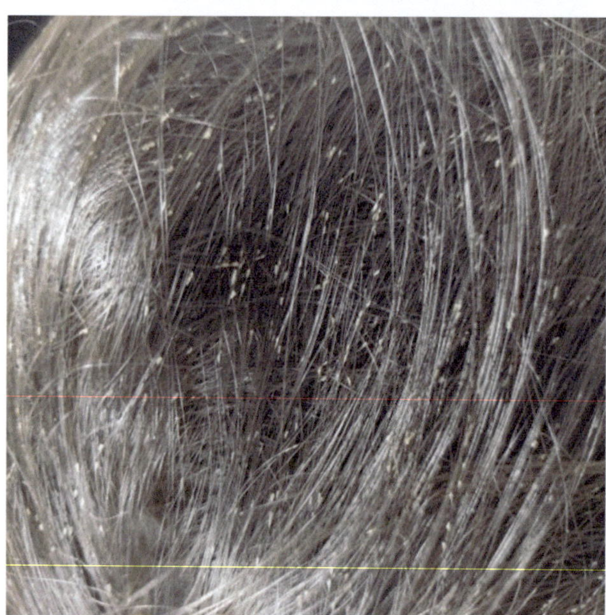

Discussion

Pediculosis capitis is a very common, highly contagious infestation caused by human head louse Pediculus Humanus Capitis. It is a very itchy condition, that can occur in anyone but children are most commonly affected. All socioeconomic

Fig. 34.3 Visible
lice on hair

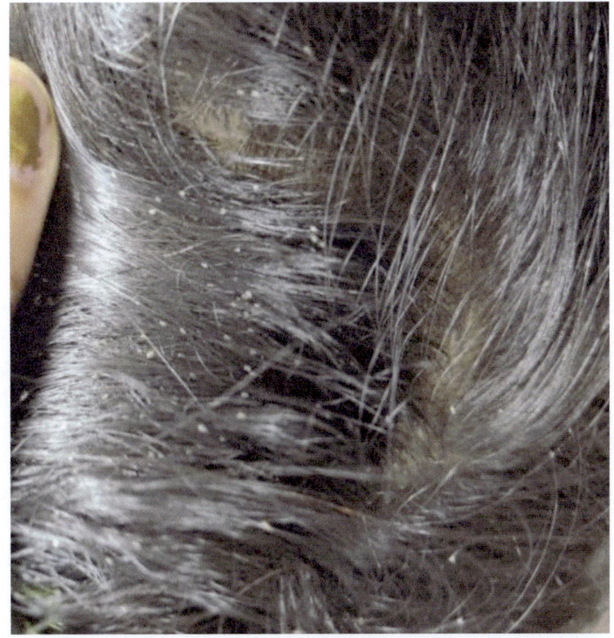

Fig. 34.4 An
eczematization on
the left eyelid

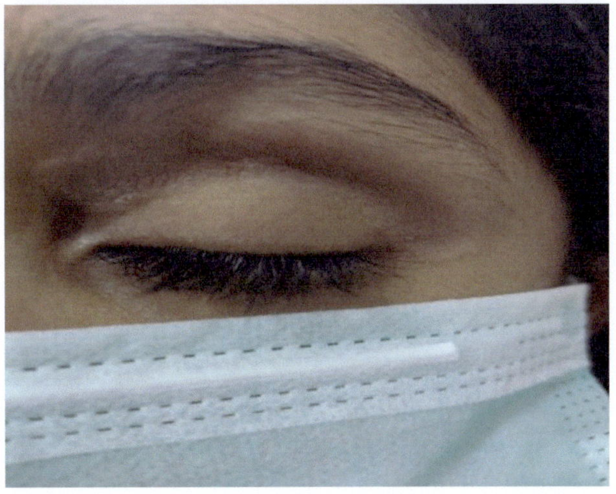

groups are at risk of pediculosis capitis. The most common symptom is continuous
itching of the scalp, neck and ears along with visible lice and nits. Anti-lice shampoo along with permethrin, malathion, lindane, crotamiton, oral ivermectin are
treatment options [1].

Pediculosis capitis can cause social distress, anxiety, irritability. It is a major
reason of embarrassment of the affected individuals. Transmission of pediculosis
capitis occurs through head to head contact and through clothing, hats, combs etc.

[2] The intensity of pruritis depends upon the duration of infestation and amount of lice present on the scalp. If not treated early it can lead to severe excoriations and due to loss of epidermal barrier secondary infections mostly caused by staphylococci and streptococci. Pediculosis capitis can lead to severe discomfort and even pain of the affected areas. Continuous scratching and chronic infestation can lead to impetinization [3]. Treatment involves manual removal of lice along with oral and topical medications. A pediculicide like permethrin, lindane etc. is prescribed not only to the patient but also to all household members. Reapplication is recommended after 10 days of the initial treatment. Oral ivermectin is also recommended [4]. The presented patient was diagnosed with pediculosis capitis. She was prescribed anti-lice shampoo, topical permethrin, oral and topical antibiotics and mild steroid for eczematization. Her mother was also asked to manually remove units. After a month she was much improved and now she is on regular follow-up.

Key Points

- Pediculosis capitis is a very common, highly contagious infestation
- It is a very itchy condition
- Anti-lice shampoo along with permethrin, malathion, lindane, crotamiton, oral ivermectin are treatment options

References

1. Janniger CK, Kuflik AS. Pediculosis capitis. Cutis. 1993;51:407–8.
2. Leung AK, Fong JH, Pinto-Rojas A. Pediculosis capitis. J Pediatr Health Care. 2005;19:369–73.
3. Solares P, Pediculosis A. Dermatol Rev Mex. 2013;57:485–90.
4. Meinking TL, Entzel P, Villar ME, Vicaria M, Lemard GA, Porcelain SL. Comparative efficacy of treatments for pediculosis capitis infestations: update 2000. Arch Dermatol. 2001;137:287–92.

Chapter 35
Presence of a Group of Hairs in Temporal Region with Different Growth Directions in Comparison with Neighboring Hairs

Nooshin Bagherani and Bruce R. Smoller

A 21-year-old man was presented with the group of hairs on the right temporal region distinguishable from the adjacent hairs by its low hair density and hair growth in different directions. The patient mentioned a patch of hair loss in the same area since birth. He underwent hair transplantation five years ago. This hair transplantation resulted in disfigurement of transplanted hairs along with their growth in different directions.

On physical examination, no abnormality in the skin texture was found within the lesion (Fig. 35.1).

Based upon the clinical feature, what is your diagnosis?

1. Woolly hair nevus.
2. Traction alopecia.
3. Triangular temporal alopecia.
4. Alopecia areata.
5. Trichotillomania.
6. Aplasia cutis congenita.

Diagnosis

Triangular temporal alopecia.

N. Bagherani (✉)
Department of Molecular Medicine, School of Advanced Technologies in Medicine, Tehran University of Medical Sciences, Tehran, Iran

B. R. Smoller
Department of Pathology and Laboratory Medicine, Department of Dermatology, University of Rochester School of Medicine and Dentistry, Rochester, NY, USA
e-mail: bruce_smoller@urmc.rochestcr.cdu

A. Waśkiel-Burnat et al. (eds.), *Clinical Cases in Hair Disorders*, Clinical Cases in Dermatology, https://doi.org/10.1007/978-3-030-93423-1_35

Fig. 35.1 A 21-year-old man complaining of area of hair growth in distinct directions disfigured growth of hairs

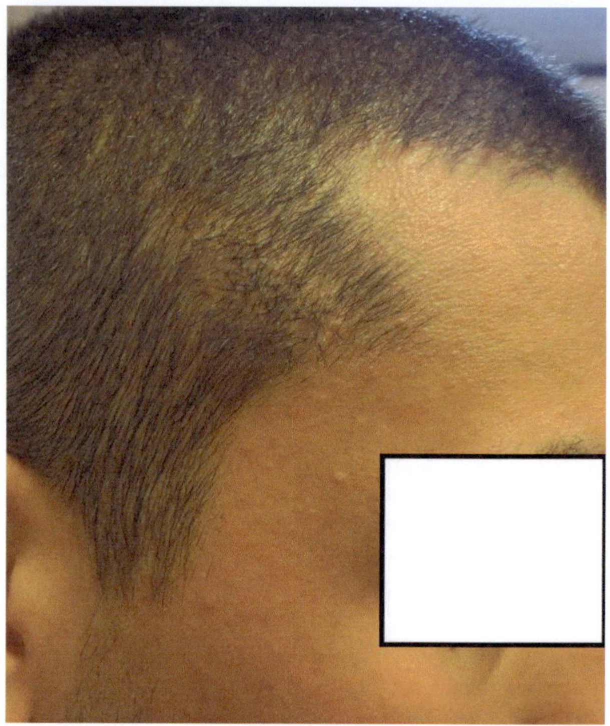

Discussion

Temporal triangular alopecia, also known as congenital triangular alopecia or Brauer nevus, is classified as benign non-cicatricial hair loss. It is characterized by an asymptomatic triangular- or oval-shaped patch of hair loss involving the temporo-parietal and occipital scalp. The lesion is often unilateral, but bilateral lesions have been reported in 20% of cases [1]. Occasionally, a few numbers of normal terminal or vellus hair can be seen within the island of hair loss [1, 2]. In some cases, instead of complete hair loss, centrally localized hair tufts or small islands of dark hairs have been reported [1]. In our case, this localized hair tuft is not a naturally occurring event, but it was secondary to prior hair transplantation.

Temporal triangular alopecia occurs at birth or during the first nine years of life and shows a nonprogressive course [3]. It shows no gender preponderance; its incidence is 0.11% in the general population [1]. The exact pathogenesis of temporal triangular alopecia is still unknown; it seems that a localized follicular miniaturization can result in this appearance [3]. A paradominant trait has been reported as its genetic bases [2].

The diagnosis of temporal triangular alopecia is mainly clinical [1, 2]. Upon pathological examination, sparse vellus hair follicles are seen replacing normal terminal hair follicles. Bone abnormalities, epilepsy, teeth abnormalities, spina bifida, woolly hair nevus, hypospadias, leukonychia, Down's syndrome, LEOPARD syndrome, Turner syndrome, and Klipple-Trenaunay syndrome are some of the disorders which have been reported in association with temporal triangular alopecia [1]. Hair restoration surgical procedures including follicular unit transplantation or surgical resection can result in satisfactory cosmetic results [1, 3].

Key Points
- Temporal triangular alopecia is classified as benign noncicatricial hair loss
- Temporal triangular alopecia appears at birth or during the first nine years of life and has a nonprogressive course
- Hair transplantation results in satisfaction of patients with temporal triangular alopecia

References

1. Yin Li VC, Yesudian PD. Congenital triangular alopecia. Int J Trichology. 2015;7(2):48–53.
2. Kelati A, Baybay H, Mernissi FZ. Temporal triangular alopecia in children: the same clinical feature for two distinct entities. Skin Appendage Disord. 2017;3(2):64–6.
3. Bang CY, Byun JW, Kang MJ, et al. Successful treatment of temporal triangular alopecia with topical minoxidil. Ann Dermatol. 2013;25(3):387–8.

Chapter 36
Single Alopecic Patches on the Scalp of Two Patients

Alejandro Martin-Gorgojo and Candida-Ana Villanueva

A 41-year-old Caucasian male with no relevant past medical history presented with a localized itch of the scalp since three years. The patient reported frequent scratching and rubbing of the area. A physical examination revealed a single, well-circumscribed, lichenified patch with short hairs, along with mild desquamation (Fig. 36.1). On dermoscopy, short hair shafts emerging from hair follicle openings and splitting distally into either smaller or equally thick tips (known as broom hairs) were observed. Moreover, white scaling was present (Fig. 36.2).

The same week, a 39 year-old Caucasian female with no relevant past medical history was evaluated for a similar lesion that had been standing for the last year (Fig. 36.3). On dermoscopy broom hairs and a small erosion were observed (Fig. 36.4).

Histology, in both patients, showed a regularly acanthotic epidermis, with no signs of spongiosis, a very sparse lymphocytic superficial perivascular infiltrate, and verticalized collagen bundles.

Based on the case description and the photographs, what is your diagnosis?

1. Seborrheic dermatitis.
2. Eczema.
3. Alopecia areata.
4. Lichen simplex chronicus.

A. Martin-Gorgojo (✉)
STI/Dermatology Department, Sección de Especialidades Médicas, Centro de Diagnóstico Médico, Madrid City Council, Madrid, Spain
e-mail: alejandromartingorgojo@aedv.es

C.-A. Villanueva
Dermatology Department, Gregorio Marañon General University Hospital, Madrid, Spain

A. Waśkiel-Burnat et al. (eds.), *Clinical Cases in Hair Disorders*, Clinical Cases in Dermatology, https://doi.org/10.1007/978-3-030-93423-1_36

Fig. 36.1 A 41-year-old man with a well-circumscribed, lichenified patch, with short hairs and mild desquamation

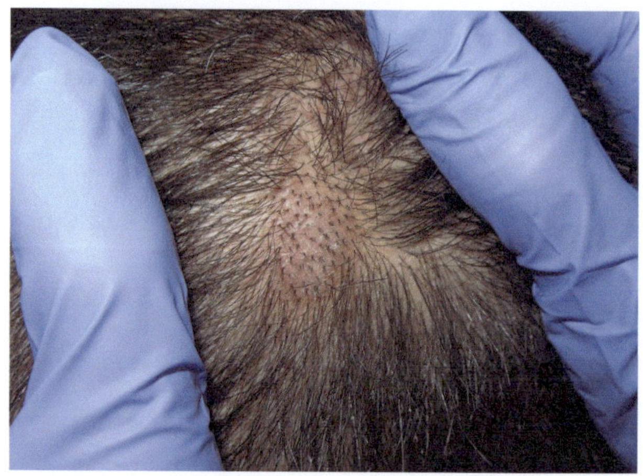

Fig. 36.2 Dermoscopy shows hair shafts emerging from hair follicle openings and splitting distally into either smaller or equally thick tips (broom hairs). Mild scaling is also present

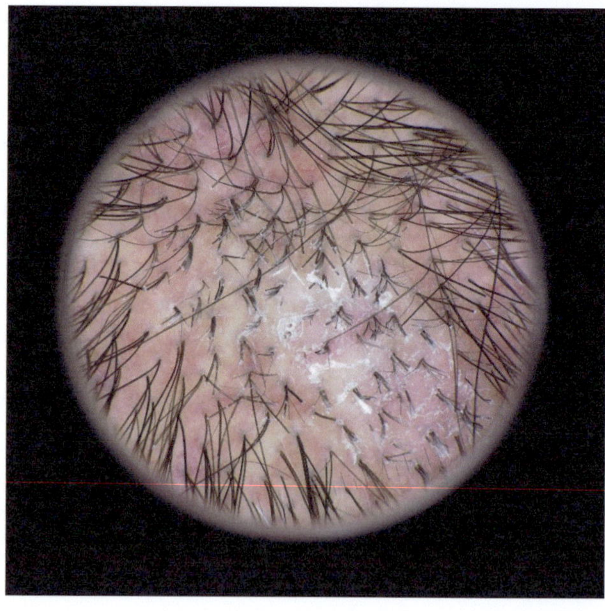

Fig. 36.3 39-year-old woman with a well-circumscribed, lichenified patch, with short hairs, and excoriation

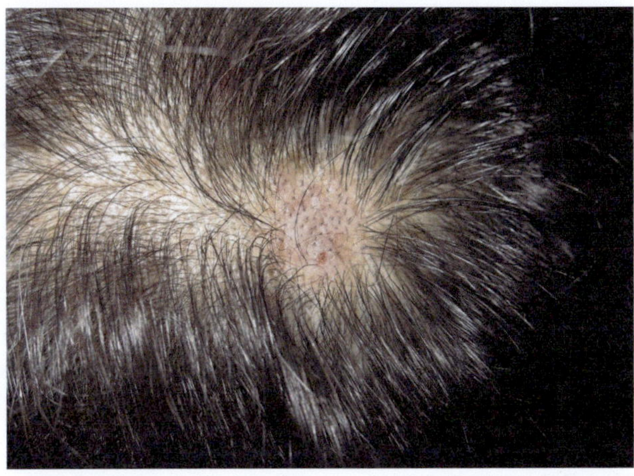

Fig. 36.4 Dermoscopy shows broom hairs and a small erosion

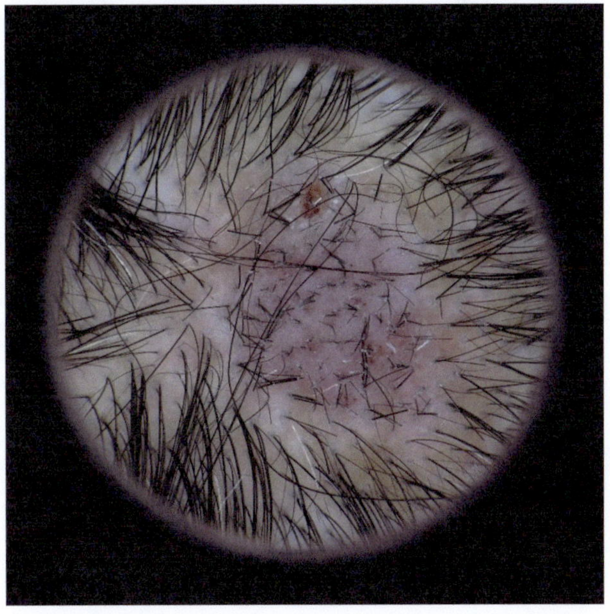

Diagnosis

Lichen simplex chronicus.

Discussion

Lichen simplex chronicus of the scalp has a characteristic dermoscopic appearance [1]. Though further diagnostic work-up may be necessary in some cases [2], the use of dermoscopy may trigger a high index of suspicion, and yield the opportunity to recommend prompt treatment, which should be preferably done with a multidisciplinary approach.

Key Points
- In case of patchy alopecia, several differential diagnosis should be taken into consideration
- Anamnesis and scalp dermoscopy (trichoscopy) are essential to identify and diagnose scalp disorders
- Certain dermoscopic and pathologic findings may yield the diagnosis of lichen simplex chronicus on the scalp

References

1. Quaresma MV, Mariño Alvarez AM, Miteva M. Dermatoscopic-pathologic correlation of lichen simplex chronicus on the scalp: 'broom fibres, gear wheels and hamburgers'. J Eur Acad Dermatol Venereol. 2016;30:343–5.
2. Ambika H, Vinod CS, Sushmita J. A case of neurodermatitis circumscipta of scalp presenting as patchy alopecia. Int J Trichology. 2013;5:94–6.

Chapter 37
Successful Treatment of Alopecia

Satya Wydya Yenny, Sigya Octari, and Heffi Anindya Putri

A seven-year-old Indonesian boy presented with a one-month history of progressively increasing areas of hair loss on the midscalp since one month (Fig. 37.1). No history of long-term medications, malignancy, hair pulling and chemotherapy was reported. The patient's father and uncle also suffered from hair loss. On physical examination, we found area of non-scarring hair loss (8 cm × 5 cm) on the midscalp. A hair pull test was negative. A trichoscopic examination revealed exclamation mark hair, black dots (cadaver hairs), yellow dots and small number of vellus hair. A direct mycological examination with potassium hydroxide did not show elements of fungi. A thyroid function was normal. Syphilis serology and antinuclear antibody tests were negative.

Based on the case description and the photographs, what is the most likely diagnosis?

1. Alopecia areata
2. Tinea capitis.
3. Alopecia syphilitica.

Based on medical history, physical examination, photograph, trichoscopy examination, and laboratory examination we diagnosed this patient with alopecia areata.

We started mometason furoate 0.1% cream in occlusion applied twice a day. The patient showed significant improvement after two months.

S. W. Yenny (✉) · S. Octari · H. A. Putri
Faculty of Medicine, Cosmetic Dermatology Division, Department of Dermatology and Venereology, Indonesian Society of Dermatology and Venereology, Dr. M. Djamil Hospital, Universitas Andalas, Padang, Indonesia
e-mail: satyawidyaycnny@med.unand.ac.id

A. Waśkiel-Burnat et al. (eds.), *Clinical Cases in Hair Disorders*, Clinical Cases in Dermatology, https://doi.org/10.1007/978-3-030-93423-1_37

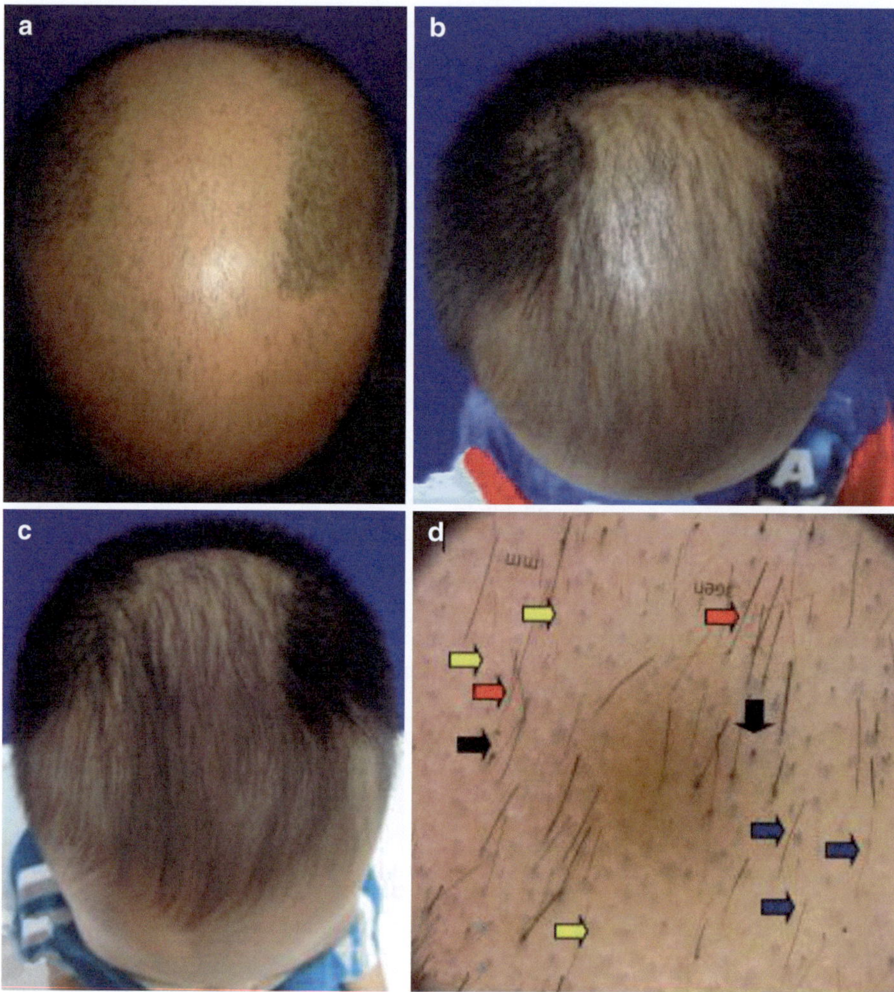

Fig. 37.1 A seven-year-old boy with patchy hair loss

Discussion

Hair loss is the most common hair growth disorder. Alopecia areata is a common autoimmune, non-scarring hair disorder that may affect any hair-bearing area. There is no sex prevalence; the incidence is higher in younger ages [1]. It is the most common form of hair loss in children [2]. Alopecia areata is characterized by an acute onset with the presence of asymptomatic, oval or round, well-circumscribed, areas of hair loss [3].

An accurate history taking is needed to determine the underlying causes of alopecia. Crucial factors include duration and pattern of hair loss, whether the hair is broken or shed at the roots, and increase of shedding or thinning. Alopecia areata may be associated with thyroid disease, syphilis, micronutrients deficiency, systemic lupus erythematosus and hereditary syndromes. Similarly to other immune-mediated diseases, a complex interplay between environment and genetics is thought to lead to the development of alopecia areata [4, 5].

Trichoscopic features of alopecia areata are exclamation mark hair, black dots, broken hair and yellow dots [6].

The Indonesian management guidelines of hair loss and alopecia recommended mild-potency topical corticosteroids as the first line therapy of alopecia areata for children under 10 years of age [2, 7].

Alopecia areata is an inflammatory disease that is caused by T cell-mediated process. Therefore therapy used to control this disease suppresses the immune response. Corticosteroids are the treatment of choice for alopecia areata, because they effectively inhibit T lymphocyte activation and help control the disease [8].

Topical corticosteroids in alopecia areata aim to reduce inflammation around and on the hair bulb, so the hair follicles can return to the normal hair cycle and give rise spontaneous resolution of alopecia [9].

The most common side effects of topical corticosteroid are folliculitis, localized skin atrophy, striae, acneiform rash, telangiectasis, dyschromia, and sometimes adrenal suppression. It is recommended to clean skin 12 hours after the application of corticosteroids to reduce the incidence of folliculitis and apply them up to five times a week to prevent atrophy [10].

Key Points
- Alopecia areata is the most common form of alopecia in children
- Trichoscopy in alopecia areata shows exclamation mark hair, black dots, broken hairs and yellow dots
- Topical corticosteroids are the first line therapy of alopecia areata in children under 10 years of age

References

1. Peloquin L, Soccio LC. Alopecia areata: an update on treatment option for children. Pediatr Drug. 2017;19:411–22.
2. Wasitaatmadja SM. Indonesian management guidelines of hair loss and alopecia. 1st ed. Wasitaatmaja SM, editor. Jakarta: Centra Communication; 2019. 32 p.
3. Alkhalifah A. Alopecia areata update. Dermatol Clin. 2013;31(1):93–108.
4. Mirzoyev SA, Schrum AG, Davis MDP, Torgerson RR. Lifetime incidence risk of alopecia areata estimated at 2.1% by Rochester Epidemiology Project, 1990-2009. J Invest Dermatol. 2014;134(4):1141–2.
5. Lee S, Lee WS. Management of alopecia areata: updates and algorithmic approach. J Dermatol. 2017:1–13.
6. Jain N, Doshi B, Khopkar U. Trichoscopy in alopecias: Diagnosis simplified. Int J Trichology. 2013;5(4):170–8.

7. Otberg N, Saphiro J. Alopecia Areata. In: Kang S, Amagam M, Brucker A, Enk AH, Margolis David J, Mcmichael AJ, et al., editors. Fitzpatricks dermatology in general medicine. 9th ed. McGraw-Hill Companies; 2019. p. 1517–22.
8. Hordinsky MK. Current treatment for alopecia areata. J Investig Dermatol Symp. 2015;17:44–6.
9. Hariani A, Jusuf NK. Evidence based treatment of alopecia areata. Berkala ilmu kesehatan kulit dan kelamin. 2017;29(2):126–34.
10. Ramos PM, Anzai A, Duque-Estrada B, Melo DF, Sternberg F, Santos LDN, Alves LD, Mulinari-Brenner F. Journal: An Bras Dermatol.

Chapter 38
The Challenge in Managing Folliculitis Decalvans

Sri Linuwih Menaldi, Eliza Miranda, Rahadi Rihatmadja, and Diah Pitaloka Prabandari

A 35-year-old male patient was referred to Dermatology and Venerology Clinic with hair loss since three years. There was a history of folliculitis and pain of the scalp. The affected area was scaly and itchy. The patient had been previously treated with ciprofloxacin and anti-dandruff shampoo with a temporary improvement. However, after treatment discontinuation the disease reccured with subsequent scarring.

On physical examination of the scalp, multiple erythematous nummular-sized macules and plaques as well as pustules, white scales, eutrophic scars, and tufted hair were presented. There was no enlargement of regional lymph nodes. A Wood's lamp examination was negative (Fig. 38.1). In microscopic examination the presence of leukocytes and Gram-positive cocci was observed. An aerobic culture showed *Enterobacter aerogenes* which was resistant to cephalothin and amoxicillin-clavulanic acid. A histopathological examination revealed epidermis within normal limits. In the dermis, there was a dense mixture of inflammatory cells consists of lymphocytes, histiocytes, polymorphonuclear leukocytes, and plasma cells.

Based on the case description and the photographs, what is your diagnosis?

1. Folliculitis decalvans.
2. Dissecting folliculitis.
3. Tinea capitis (kerion).

S. L. Menaldi (✉) · E. Miranda · R. Rihatmadja · D. P. Prabandari
Faculty of Medicine, Department of Dermatology and Venereology, Indonesian Society of Dermatology and Venereology, Universitas Indonesia/Dr. Cipto Mangunkusumo National Central General Hospital, Jakarta, Indonesia

A. Waśkiel-Burnat et al. (eds.), *Clinical Cases in Hair Disorders*, Clinical Cases in Dermatology, https://doi.org/10.1007/978-3-030-93423-1_38

Fig. 38.1 Scarring
alopecia with the presence
of tufted hair

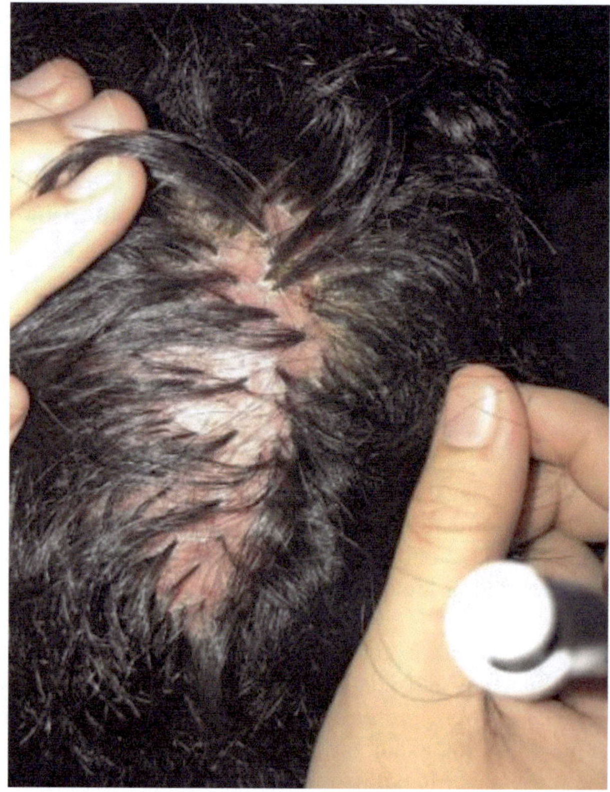

Diagnosis

Folliculitis decalvans.

Discussion

Folliculitis decalvans is an inflammatory disease characterized by pustular folliculitis on the scalp. The disease leads to hair loss and scarring alopecia [1, 2]. Tufted hair is characteristic feature [2]. Differential diagnoses for folliculitis decalvans included tinea capitis and dissecting cellulitis. In the presented patient, tinea capitis was excluded based on the negative examination with Wood's lamp and a mycological examination. Histology showed the features of folliculitis decalvans excluding the diagnosis of dissecting cellulitis.

The aim of the therapy of folliculitis decalvans is to avoid relapses and further damage of hair follicles as well as to treat scarring alopecia. Treatment of folliculitis decalvans include mainly topical and systemic antibiotics. To reduce an inflammation, topical and intralesional corticosteroids may be useful [3]. Systemic retinoids should be considered in case of prolonged relapses [4]. Hair transplantation shows various results [5].

The presented patient was diagnosed with folliculitis decalvans. He received intralesional injections of corticosteroids every two weeks in addition to topical fusidic acid. Three months after the treatment initiation, a partial improvement was observed. The patient was started with 20 mg of oral isotretinoin three times per week for three months. The dose of isotretinoin was decreased because of severe dryness of the skin and lips. A limited number of pustular lesions persisted.

Key Points
- Folliculitis decalvans is a form of scarring alopecia
- Tufted hair is characteristic feature of folliculitis decalvans
- The aim of the therapy of folliculitis decalvans is to avoid relapses and further damage of hair follicles as well as to treat scarring alopecia

References

1. Otberg N, Shapiro J. Cicatricial alopecias. In: Kang S, Amagai M, Bruckner AL, Enk AH, Morgolis DJ, McMichael AJ, et al., editors. Fitzpatrick's dermatology. 9th ed. McGraw-Hill Education; 2019. p. 1524–36.
2. Annessi G. Tufted folliculitis of the scalp: a distinctive clinicohistological variant of folliculitis decalvans. Br J Dermatol. 1998;138(5):799–805.
3. Pimenta R, Borges-Costa J. Successful treatment with fusidic acid in a patient with folliculitis decalvans. Acta Dermatovenerol Croat. 2019;27(1):49–50.
4. Tietze JK, Heppt MV, von Preußen A, et al. Oral isotretinoin as the most effective treatment in folliculitis decalvans: a retrospective comparison of different treatment regimens in 28 patients. J Eur Acad Dermatol Venereol. 2015;29(9):1816–21.
5. Ekelem C, Pham C, Atanaskova MN. A systematic review of the outcome of hair transplantation in primary scarring alopecia. Skin Appendage Disord. 2019;5(2):65–71.

Index

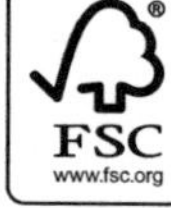

MIX
Papier aus verantwortungsvollen Quellen
Paper from responsible sources
FSC® C105338

If you have any concerns about our products,
you can contact us on
ProductSafety@springernature.com

In case Publisher is established outside the EU,
the EU authorized representative is:
Springer Nature Customer Service Center GmbH
Europaplatz 3, 69115 Heidelberg, Germany

Printed by Libri Plureos GmbH
in Hamburg, Germany